Foods That Fight Disease

Laurie Deutsch Mozian, M.S., R.D.

Foods That

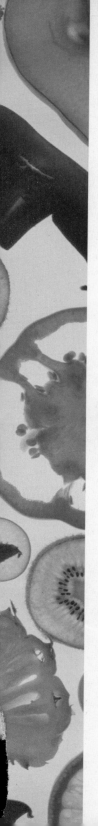

Fight Disease

*A Simple Guide to
Using and Understanding
Phytonutrients to Protect and
Enhance Your Health*

Avery
a member of
Penguin Putnam Inc.

Every effort has been made to ensure that the information contained in this book is complete and accurate. However, neither the publisher nor the author is engaged in rendering professional advice or services to the individual reader. The ideas, procedures, and suggestions contained in this book are not intended as a substitute for consulting with your physician. All matters regarding health require medical supervision. Neither the author nor the publisher shall be liable or responsible for any loss, injury, or damage allegedly arising from any information or suggestion in this book.

Most Avery books are available at special quantity discounts for bulk purchase for sales promotions, premiums, fund-raising, and educational needs. Special books or book excerpts also can be created to fit specific needs. For details, write Putnam Special Markets, 375 Hudson Street, New York, NY 10014.

Avery
a member of
Penguin Putnam Inc.
375 Hudson Street
New York, NY 10014
www.penguinputnam.com

Library of Congress Cataloging-in-Publication Data

Mozian, Laurie Deutsch.
    Foods that fight disease : a simple guide to using and understanding phytonutrients
  to protect and enhance your health/Laurie Deutsch Mozian.
        p.   cm.
    Includes bibliographical references and index.
    ISBN 1-58333-037-2
    1. Functional foods.   2. Nutrition   3. Phytochemicals.   I. Title.
  [DNLM: 1. Food.   2. Nutritive value.   3. Plant physiology.
  4. Plants—chemistry. 5. Plants—metabolism.]
  RA784.M69   2000   00-025647
  613.2—dc21

Printed in the United States of America
10   9   8   7   6   5   4   3   2   1

Book design by Lee Fukui

In loving memory of Violette Strauss Deutsch, Gertrude Resnikoff Strauss, and Marie Lombardi Horan

Credits

Table 1.1 on page 14 is reprinted with permission from the *Journal of Agricultural and Food Chemistry*, vol. 42, no. 8 (1994). Copyright © 1994 American Chemical Society.

Table 1.2 on page 15 is reprinted with permission from the *Journal of Alternative and Complementary Medicine*, vol. 3, no. 1 (1997): 7–12.

Table 3.1 on page 34 is adapted from *Nutrition Action Health Letter* (1875 Connecticut Ave., N.W., Suite 300, Washington, D.C. 20009-5728. $24.00 for 10 issues.) Copyright © 1998 CSPI

Table 3.2 on page 40 is reprinted with permission from Dr. Connie Weaver and *The Soy Connection Newsletter*.

Table 3.3 on page 46 is reprinted with permission from *Journal of Agricultural and Food Chemistry* 45 (1997): 3076–3082. Copyright © 1997 American Chemical Society.

Table 4.1 on page 92 is reprinted with permission from the Indiana Soybean Board.

The "Sweet Maple Nuggets" recipe on page 203 is adapted from a recipe from the Indiana Soybean Board. Used with permission.

Acknowledgments

My deepest thanks go to my husband, Paul, whose love and generosity of spirit are infectious—he enables all the members of our family to work toward their potential; to Rudy Shur for his vision—he saw a book where once there was none; to Dara Stewart, who gently guided my research and words into a book; and to Mary Jo Russell, the crackerjack medical librarian at Vassar Brothers Hospital in Poughkeepsie, New York, for her extraordinary and cheerful efforts on my behalf.

I depended on personal communications with many scientists in order for them to explain their research to me. I am grateful to Dr. H. Leon Bradlow from Strang Cornell Research Laboratories in New York City and Dr. Charles Elson from the University of Wisconsin at Madison for the time and assistance they gave me. I want to thank Dr. James Duke, Dr. John Potter, Dr. Stephen Hecht, Dr. Connie Weaver, Dr. Pam Crowell, Dr. Lisa Brown, Dr. Lee W. Wattenberg, and Dr. Winston Craig for responding to my questions.

I could not have completed this project without a remarkably flexible work schedule. Special thanks to my coworkers, particularly Barbara Saintomas, for making this possible.

My thanks to Judy Fischetti at the Woodstock Library for her help, to Ellen Messer for her kindness and her lesson in publishing tenacity, and to Robin Berger for being my first reader.

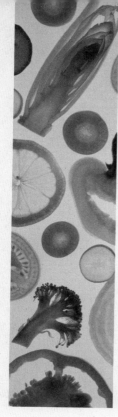

Contents

Preface

The seed for this book was planted many years ago at a kitchen table in Queens, New York, by a chance remark made by my mother's friend. We were discussing salad ingredients, and she said, "Don't waste time eating cucumbers. They have nothing to offer in the way of nourishment." I don't remember responding, but a little voice in my head told me that everything that grows has some value and sustains us in some way. My explorations into the intricacies of phytochemicals have offered me validation for my theory.

Predictably, I went on to choose a career in nutrition. No one selects this area of study to become rich and famous. I chose my profession because I truly believe that what I do is important. So imagine my delight when I saw a headline in the *New York Times* in 1994 that read, "Benefits of Broccoli Confirmed as Chemical Blocks Tumor." I hung this article on the refrigerator right next to the one from 1992 that said a chemical in celery lowers blood pressure. These were soon joined by another *New York Times* clipping that read, "Tomatoes Found to Reduce Risk of Cancer." Eventually, I had to buy a file box to hold all my clippings, and I felt the idea for a book begin to stir inside me.

Since I had never undertaken a project quite as prodigious as this before, the process itself has been exhilarating. Sometimes it seemed self-propelled, and other times it needed my administration. Attempting to master the process has been more challenging than acquiring the information that goes between the covers.

My goal in writing this book was to make this science available for both laypeople and professionals alike. I particularly wanted to make the information about the physical mechanisms that foods stimulate accessible to health professionals so they might gain a greater respect for and understanding of the roles that specific foods play in health and healing. I hope this book proves to be a useful guide to those people who are seeking to change their diets to enhance the quality of their lives.

Introduction

Imagine you were given the job of designing the perfect medicine. How would it work? Would it accomplish its task and leave the body with as few negative side effects as possible? How about if it came in a brightly colored package that was also biodegradable? It's too late. It has already been done. The package is food, and the medicine is phytochemicals.

Phytochemicals are found in all plant life. *Phyto-* comes from the Greek word for plant. Frequently, phytochemicals act as one would hope the perfect drug would act. They effect positive change in the body without leaving behind any harmful side effects. The varying amounts of phytochemicals in a particular food are responsible for its color and taste. We are learning that phytochemicals also are responsible for the food's ability to impede the disease process. Certain foods may be suitable for targeting certain diseases because of their phyto-chemical makeup.

For many years, we've known that people who eat more whole grains, fruits, and vegetables have less disease. We know this from ex-amining the diets of different populations around the world. However, until recently, we didn't know exactly why. We had assumed that the low fat and high fiber content of their diets conferred health benefits. But this is just part of the truth. Another part of the picture of the way foods help fight disease is emerging, and it includes the existence of phytochemicals in our foods that previously were unknown to us. The knowledge we are gaining about phytochemicals will change the way we eat in both sickness and health.

The typical standard American diet is heavily based on animal foods, white flour, and sugar, and we are plagued with high rates of heart disease, cancer, high blood pressure, and diabetes. The problem that exists as a result of our getting the bulk of our calories from ani-mal foods and refined grains might be twofold. Not only are we taking in an excessive amount of fat and sugar, but we are also taking in a de-creased amount of phytochemicals. Dr. John Potter, a scientist at the Fred Hutchinson Cancer Research Center in Seattle, Washington, has been investigating the relationship between diet and disease for twenty years. He has concluded, "We're running our engines on the wrong bi-ological fuel."

As a nutritionist, I am often confronted with sickness and asked, "Is there anything I can eat that will help?" For years, we've known that vegetarians were healthier, but we didn't really know why. With in-creased knowledge about the way foods and phytochemicals work in the body, we can better design diets that can precisely pinpoint our special needs. This book will provide you with a clear understanding of what phytochemicals do and in which foods they can be found.

Food is a medicine you can use without a prescription. Phyto-chemicals put the ability to fight disease in your hands. Along with a healthy diet, certain phytochemicals may be useful in preventing and treating cancer, diabetes, heart disease, menopause, premenstrual syn-drome, osteoporosis, prostate problems, and a number of other dis-eases. The message is a positive one—the addition of certain foods to your diet will help you to fight disease. The statement made in 1918 by the famous biochemist and professor of nutrition E. V. McCollum, "Eat what you want after you eat what you should," continues to hold true.

The phytochemicals found in foods might be the most exciting nutrition information uncovered in the last half of the twentieth century. Some of these phytochemicals can actually travel to the DNA of the cell and protect it from being changed by carcinogens that enter the body and ultimately lead to cancer. Some phytochemicals stifle blood-vessel formation that is needed to bring a developing tumor the nutrients it needs to grow. Some alter hormone production. Some phytochemicals, like those in fiber, may act in a mechanical fashion, creating pressure and speeding the movement of food through the body. With knowledge about how phytochemicals work to prevent disease comes the concept of chemoprevention—preventing specific diseases by increasing exposure to certain phytochemicals that produce the desired effect.

This book will tell you not only what phytochemicals in foods can do but also how to include more of them in the framework of a healthy diet. A professor of mine once said, "It's easier for people to change their language than to change their eating habits." She pointed out that in every ethnic neighborhood, an ethnic grocery store still offers residents familiar foods even after they have adopted English as their language. With that in mind, remember, all change is a process. Changing your diet means more than changing your food; it can mean changing your life. When you make forward motion to start eating healthier fare, you are not only reducing your disease risk, you are empowering yourself. You are taking responsibility for your health. You are passing on a legacy of good eating habits to your family.

This book also includes recipes for families in transition from a meat-based diet to a plant-based diet. As a mother, I know how frustrating and time consuming it can be to prepare a healthy meal and have your family turn up their noses at it and leave the table hungry because the food is unfamiliar. Therefore, I include recipes that mix the familiar with the unfamiliar so the family can be introduced to new foods in a nonthreatening way. Consider every new phytochemical-rich food you introduce into your meals a victory for good health.

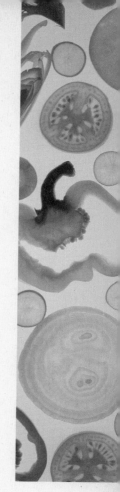

Part I

All About Phytochemicals

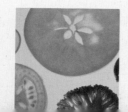

What is all this talk about phytochemicals? How will they help me prevent disease? Why should I include more of them in my diet? I'm sure these questions go through people's minds every day. We often hear about including more vitamins and minerals in our diets, but rarely do we hear about phytochemicals. Before I tell you which phytochemicals are best for preventing which diseases, you need to know what phytochemicals are and how they work in the body. Part One of this book will give you all that information and more.

1

What Are Phytochemicals?

 What makes an orange orange? What accounts for its distinctive aroma? The answer to both questions is the same—phytochemicals. But phytochemicals do more than just color and flavor food. Phytochemicals are biologically active nonnutritive substances that appear in all plant foods (*phyto-* comes from the Greek word for plant). They are responsible for giving plants their color, flavor, and disease resistance. Each bite of fruit, vegetable, or whole grain you eat is packed with hundreds of phytochemicals. Many phytochemicals appear to have a major impact upon your health. Most are fat-free and calorie-free, and though they are not considered essential for health, your life might depend upon them. Worldwide, chemists are studying phytochemicals to determine their potential to prevent and fight disease in people. Phytochemicals are the new frontier in nutrition.

PHYTOCHEMICALS—NUTRIENTS OR DRUGS?

When considering the activities of phytochemicals, the question arises—Are phytochemicals foods or drugs? According to Dr. John Pinto, the director of the Nutrition Research Laboratory of Sloan-Kettering Memorial Hospital in New York City, "When phytochemicals are consumed in excess of the quantity that can be obtained from food—the line between food and drug is crossed and phytochemicals are being used as pharmaceuticals."

Phytonutrients

Under the umbrella term "phytochemicals" falls a subset of nutritive plant chemicals, called phytonutrients—biologically active plant substances that have been determined to be necessary to sustain life—in other words, vitamins and minerals found in plants. Ascorbic acid (the plant form of vitamin C) is an example of a phytonutrient. Unlike phytochemicals, phytonutrients have been determined to be necessary to promote life, and Recommended Dietary Allowances have been established for them by the National Academy of Science. We know how much phytonutrient intake is sufficient to ward off certain diseases. However, science has yet to determine the specific quantities we need of many phytochemicals to keep disease away.

Nutraceuticals and Pharmafoods

"Nutraceutical" and "pharmafood" are words that meld nutrients with pharmaceuticals in an effort to describe a food's ability to act as both a nutrient and a drug. Nutraceuticals and pharmafoods are any substance that may be considered a food or part of a food and that provides medical or health benefits, including the prevention and treatment of disease. Perillyl alcohol, found in cherries, is an example of a nutraceutical. Derived from fruit, a source of nutrition, perillyl alcohol is being evaluated for its potential as an anticancer pharmaceutical.

Regardless of how we define these food components or what we call them, it's clear that we need to understand how phytochemicals affect our bodies so that we can select an optimal diet.

HOW PHYTOCHEMICALS WORK

Phytochemicals, those powerful disease-fighting molecules that are buried in the very matrix of the food we eat, work in a variety of ways. Some act as antioxidants, some stimulate enzyme systems, and some alter hormone production. Some phytochemicals serve as raw material for the body's production of its own anticancer substances, some detoxify cancer-causing substances by binding or diluting carcinogens, and some deflect the activation of cancer-causing substances. Their methods of action often overlap and assist one another. Some phytochemicals can work to both prevent and suppress the disease process.

When it comes to the methods that phytochemicals employ to protect us from disease, there is a great deal of repetition of mechanisms. Many different foods offer the same phytochemicals. For instance, the phytochemical limonene appears in citrus fruits and in spices. In addition, many different phytochemicals use identical methods to intervene with disease processes. Curcumin, which is found in the spice turmeric, and ascorbic acid, which is found in citrus fruits, both block the formation of nitrosamines, cancer-causing compounds.

Frequently, a food will contain a multitude of phytochemicals from many chemical families, each with a variety of activities. Although chemists examine each phytochemical for the specific benefits it contributes, it is possible that the true value of phytochemicals comes in the interaction, or the synergy, among them.

Stimulating Enzymes Both Good and Bad

Some phytochemicals act by stimulating various enzyme systems in the body. There are multitudes of enzyme systems, which perform in a variety of ways. One rather complex enzyme system that phyochemicals stimulate is the phase I cytochrome p450 enzyme system. This system activates or detoxifies certain cancer-causing agents. Some scientists are concerned with the aftermath of stimulating this system. Other scientists claim that the net effect of stimulating this mixed-function system is less cancer, so they see no cause for worry.

When stimulated, this enzyme system triggers the release of the enzyme cytochrome p450 in the cell. This is where things get tricky—sometimes cytochrome p450 detoxifies cancer-causing substances, and sometimes it activates them, depending upon the specific cancer-causing substances present. The net effect of stimulating the mixed-function system appears to be a benefit rather than a detriment.

Other phytochemicals appear to stimulate the phase II enzyme system. It is more desirable that this enzyme system be stimulated than the mixed-function system because its enzymes work to encourage the transformation of cancer-causing agents into harmless substances. Glutathione-S-transferase (GST) is a phase II enzyme whose activity is increased by certain phytochemicals found in foods. Glutathione-S-transferase stimulates an increased tissue level of the cellular antioxidant glutathione, which is made from the amino acid glutamine. (An antioxidant is a substance that combats the damaging effects of free radicals—harmful molecules that circulate the body looking to steal an electron from other molecules.) Glutathione is a carrier of amino acids into the

Stimulating GST in Different Parts of the Body

Many different phytochemicals stimulate increased glutathione-S-transferase (GST) activity, but the phytochemicals from some foods appear to favor increased GST in certain organs in the body. For example, the diallyl sulfides that are found in onions and garlic dramatically and consistently increase the levels of GST in the stomach, whereas the dithiolethiones found in cruciferous vegetables also increase GST levels, but not necessarily in the stomach. This helps support the belief that an increased risk of certain cancers or exposure to substances that are known to cause certain cancers might be offset by an increased intake of certain phytochemicals that deliver a desired effect.

cell and a cellular scavenger of free radicals. It protects the cellular DNA from damage. It is enzyme-mediated, which means that you can only get more glutathione in the cell by stimulating the enzymes that catalyze it, like glutathione-S-transferase (GST).

Glutathione-S-transferase works in the cell to block carcinogens from reaching the DNA by promoting the union of carcinogens with glutathione to form less toxic substances and more water-soluble substances that can be easily excreted from the body. In this way, glutathione-S-transferase scuttles carcinogens out of the body before they reach and damage the cell's DNA.

Since phytochemicals do not appear singularly in foods but rather in groups, often when a food contains a phytochemical that stimulates the mixed-function enzyme system, it has other phytochemicals that stimulate phase II enzymes. In this way, the phytochemicals work together as parallel lines of defense to offer protection against disease.

Phytochemicals as Antioxidants

Phytochemicals that act as antioxidants offer protection against disease through their ability to quench hungry free-radical molecules that are created in the body in the course of normal metabolism. Free radicals are excited singular molecules that travel among the cells and the cell membranes looking for a molecule to pair up with. If they do not find it readily, they will steal it from a cell, setting off a chain reaction that can lead to damaged DNA and the genesis of disease. The presence of an ample supply of antioxidants in the cell and the cell membrane helps to ensure the integrity of the cell and saves it from damage by free-radical molecules. In simplistic terms, think of free radicals as roving gangs of thug molecules, looking to start trouble in the cell, and the antioxidants as martyrs, who offer themselves as sacrifices, saving the cell from attack. We need more than one type of antioxidant in our diet because some antioxidants function best in the cell membrane, which is an oil-based environment, and some work in the interior of the cell, which is water-based.

The antioxidant properties of phytochemicals and phytonutrients

> ## ORAC: A New Value for Assessing the Antioxidant Capacity of Food
>
> Scientists at the United States Department of Agriculture (USDA) measure the antioxidant ability of foods to subdue oxygen free radicals in test tubes. The value used to express this ability is called its Oxygen Radical Absorbance Capacity (ORAC). Thus far, foods with high ORAC activity, such as spinach, strawberries, and blueberries, have raised the antioxidant power of human blood. Scientists say that the increases in plasma ORAC can't be explained fully by increases in levels of the separate antioxidant vitamins. They theorize that the body must be absorbing other compounds from fruits and vegetables. (Might these "other compounds" be the up-and-coming phytochemicals?)

described above appear to be imperative in the prevention of cancer and cardiovascular disease.

Preventing Nitrosamine Production

Some phytochemicals offer disease protection by preventing the activation of nitrosamines in the stomach. Nitrosamines are cancer-causing substances that are created by a combination of nitrites with amines that have been activated to cause cancer. Nitrites commonly are found in nature and can be in the food and water supply. Increased exposure can come from processed foods that are treated with nitrites. Phytochemicals can act to block the activation and subsequent metamorphosis of nitrosamines into their cancer-causing state.

Impeding Cholesterol Production

Some phytochemicals have the potential to suppress tumor growth and modestly decrease cholesterol levels by interfering with the pathway that leads to cholesterol production. HMG-COA reductase is a raw material needed by cells to synthesize cholesterol and encourage tumor growth. Some phytochemicals interfere with the HMG-COA reductase pathway and therefore suppress tumor cell reproduction and the accumulation of cholesterol.

CLASSES OF PHYTOCHEMICALS

Though there are hundreds of different phytochemicals, several of them are similar in function or composition and are thus grouped into categories. Following are some of those phytochemical families.

Carotenoids

Carotenoids are a family of over 450 phytochemicals that includes beta-carotene and lycopene. Carotenoids are powerful antioxidants that stabilize free radicals in the cell membrane. Some carotenoids also serve as precursors to vitamin A. Carotenoids deflect oxidative damage in the cell and appear to help protect against heart disease and certain cancers. Availability of carotenoids for absorption is influenced by heat and particle size. With optimal heating—enough heat to cook but not overcook—carotenoids increase in bioavailability. Carotenoids are found in most green leafy vegetables and red-orange fruits and vegetables.

Isoflavones

Isoflavones are phytochemicals that are found chiefly in beans. The best studied of the isoflavones are genistein and daidzein. High quantities of isoflavones are found in soybeans and soy products, as well as other legumes. They also are found in kudzu and red clover, plants that are edible but seldom used as foods. Tables 1.1 and 1.2 indicate the amount of isoflavones found in a variety of foods.

Isoflavones have the power to inhibit cancer growth in a number of ways. The isoflavone genistein has been noted to inhibit angiogenesis, the birth of new blood vessels. New blood vessels must grow into a tumor in order for that tumor to spread. The tumor sends out signals to stimulate the growth of these new blood vessels, which serve as road-

Table 1.1. Amount of Isoflavones Found in Soy Foods

Food	Amount of Isoflavones in 3.5 Ounces
Roasted soybeans	162.5 mg
Textured soy protein	138.2 mg
Green soybeans	135.4 mg
Soy flour	112.4 mg
Tempeh	62.5 mg
Tofu	33.7 mg
Tofu yogurt	16.4 mg
Soy hot dog	15.0 mg
Soymilk	9.65 mg
Soy noodles (dry)	8.5 mg

ways for the cancer to travel to the rest of the body. Genistein inhibits the tumor's ability to engage in angiogenesis. It is interesting to note that angiogenesis is not an everyday occurrence. It happens infrequently during the life cycle—in the process of wound healing, during pregnancy, and in the progression of cancer.

In Japan, where about 200 milligrams of isoflavones are consumed per day on average, men demonstrate a very low mortality rate from prostate cancer, although the incidence of in situ prostate cancer (tumors that never developed blood vessels and thus were never able to advance) upon autopsy is similar to that of men in Western societies. It is thought that the high levels of genistein in the blood inhibits the in situ tumor from developing blood vessels to spread to other parts of the body.

On average, Asians in Asia consume 1.5 to 2 milligrams of soy isoflavones per kilogram of body weight per day. It is assumed that proportional quantities of isoflavones would confer the same protection against cancer we see in Asian countries. To determine how much you will need, divide your weight by 2.2 and multiply that figure by 1.75. According to those figures, a 150-pound woman would need to take in 102 to 136 milligrams of isoflavones daily to reach a therapeutic dose.

Isoflavones as Phytoestrogens

Isoflavones also have the ability to act as weak estrogens, so they are often referred to as phytoestrogens, which means plant estrogens. Genistein and daidzein, the major isoflavones found largely in legumes and soy products, lead to the production of equol in people and some animals. Equol is a weak estrogen possessing about 0.2 percent of the biological activity of estradiol, one of the major estrogens found in the body. Depending upon a person's own estrogen production and the tissue in question, the weak estrogenic effects of isoflavones can either hinder or enhance the action of natural estrogens in the body. Phytoestrogens are thought to compete with the body's own estrogen for attachment to the estrogen receptors, which are on the outside of estrogen-sensitive cells,

Table 1.2. The Amount of Isoflavones Found in Various Seeds

Food	Genistein (milligrams per 100 grams)	Daidzein (milligrams per 100 grams)
Kudzu root	316 mg	949 mg
Yellow split peas	45 mg	0.4 mg
Black turtle beans	45 mg	0.4 mg
Baby lima beans	40 mg	0.4 mg
Large lima beans	34 mg	0.3 mg
Anasazi beans	30 mg	6.5 mg
Red kidney beans	29 mg	2.7 mg
Red lentils	25 mg	5.2 mg
Soybeans	24 mg	37 mg
Black-eyed peas	23 mg	0.3 mg
Pinto beans	22 mg	23 mg
Mung beans	22 mg	0.3 mg
Adzuki beans	21 mg	4.6 mg
Fava beans	20 mg	5.0 mg
Great Northern beans	18 mg	7.2 mg

thus diminishing the amount of genuine estrogen that enters the cell. They serve to block the uptake of the body's own estrogen and environmental estrogens. In this way, phytoestrogens may act as inhibitors of hormone-dependent cancers (breast, cervical, and endometrial), which are fueled by estrogen.

Isoflavones also have the ability to inhibit cancers that are not hormone dependent through another mechanism. The isoflavone genistein acts specifically as an inhibitor of the enzyme tyrosine kinase. Tyrosine kinase appears to activate the growth of tumor cells and encourages the aggregation of blood platelets, which leads to blockages in the cardiovascular system. This suggests the isoflavone genistein would be useful in inhibiting both cancer and cardiovascular disease. In an animal study, prostate tumors that were transplanted into animals whose diets were supplemented with isoflavones failed to manifest.

Isoflavones and Bone Density

Short-term studies of postmenopausal women have indicated that a higher concentration of isoflavones in the diet may lead to increased density of the lower spine. This may be due to the estrogenic effects of the isoflavone genistein. After menopause, women have decreased amounts of circulating estrogen. It is believed that estrogen helps women maintain bone density. The decreases in estrogen levels that occur after menopause are thought to lead to increased bone loss, which can precipitate osteoporosis. The isoflavone genistein, which is present in legumes, has the ability to bind almost entirely with an estrogen receptor present on the cell membrane. This might explain genistein's ability to prevent bone loss in rats that have had their ovaries removed and have no source of estrogen. For women with low levels of estrogen, isoflavones might act as an estrogen replacement and thus promote stronger bones.

Isoflavones and the Symptoms of Menopause

Asian women who follow a typical Asian lifestyle do not complain of the symptoms of menopause, such as night sweats, hot flashes, and vaginal dryness, that their American counterparts do. It is thought that they might be protected by their high dietary intake of isoflavones due to the high soy content of their diet. The ability of isoflavones to imitate some of the beneficial effects of estrogen might explain this discrepancy between American and Asian women. To learn if diet can impact the symptoms of menopause, a few studies that tested the effects of increasing dietary isoflavones have resulted in conflicting findings. Some studies have shown a 40-percent decrease in incidence and intensity of hot flashes with the addition of 45 grams of soy foods to the diet in six weeks. Other studies have not found any decrease in hot flashes but have detected an increase in the amount of cells in the vagina, which can prevent the thinning of the vaginal wall, vaginal dryness, and pain during intercourse that some postmenopausal women experience.

Isoflavone Intake in Childhood

Isoflavone intake is as important for children as it is for adults. You can affect your children's risk of developing cancer later in life by what you feed them now. According to Dr. Stephen Barnes, a well-known cancer researcher, "Early life exposure to phytoestrogens has lifelong effects. The cells that lead to cancer are laid down during the teen years, but until those cells form a tumor, you don't have cancer."

Isoflavones and Diabetes

The isoflavone genistein works as a tyrosine kinase inhibitor. Tyrosine kinase is an enzyme that acts as an intracellular messenger, and the message it carries appears to contribute to the premature development of cardiovascular disease—a complication of diabetes. People with diabetes develop the clogged arteries that lead to cardiovascular disease at an earlier age than average for the general population. High blood sugar induces proteins in the interior of the cell to send a message to the cell membrane to attract molecules that are adhesive and will cause blood cell coagulation in the arteries. Increased intake of isoflavones through increased legume consumption might help reduce the increased activity of tyrosine kinase, which contributes to excessive deposits in the arteries.

Isoprenoids

Isoprenoids battle cancer in two ways. Like many other phytochemicals found in vegetables, they increase the phase II enzyme glutathione-S-transferase, and thus diffuse the potential of cancer-causing substances before they damage the DNA of the cell. In addition, they have a unique mechanism that protects the cancer cell from reproducing. Isoprenoids are phytochemical constituents of many plant foods. It is estimated that there are 22,000 isoprenoid compounds in the plant world. The monoterpene phytochemicals (see page 19) found in citrus fruits and cherries, geraniol found in carrots, and the tocotrienols found in whole grains have isoprenoid activity.

In order to understand the mechanism by which isoprenoids work, you must first know a little about how cells work. Most cells have feedback mechanisms that help them attract the molecules they need to do their work and repel those same molecules when they are present in abundance. This feedback system works in a similar fashion to the thirst mechanism. When you are thirsty, you crave water. When you have enough water and are sated, you are no longer thirsty and would refuse that same water if it were offered.

This feedback mechanism is faulty in cancer cells—cancer cells never signal the body that they have enough cholesterol, so the cells keep making mevalonate, the raw material needed to create cholesterol. Mevalonate's products synthesize HMG-COA reductase. Cancer cells are overloaded with HMG-COA reductase. This HMG-COA reductase makes the cells more tumor-friendly and encourages them to reproduce. The isoprenoid phytochemicals degrade the HMG-COA reductase and impair it from working, thus decreasing the ability of the cancer cell to reproduce. According to Dr. Charles Elson, who researches the effects in the body of isoprenoids from foods at the University of Wisconsin, the drug Mevacor (lovastatin), which is used to treat cancer and heart disease, works on this mechanism, but Mevacor stops all cells from dividing, not just the tumor cells, whereas iso-prenoid phytochemicals work selectively on tumor cells.

It is estimated that 500 milligrams of isoprenoid would provide a chemopreventive dose. The normal diet of a vegetarian or of a person who gets most of their calories from plant foods would supply close to 500 milligrams of isoprenoid phytochemicals. Experts predict that more isoprenoids would be necessary to provide a therapeutic dose.

Isothiocynates

Isothiocynates are a family of phytochemicals that induces protective phase II enzymes, thus making them protective against cancer. Sulfora-phane, benzyl isothiocynate, and phenyl ethyl isothiocynate (PEITC) are members of the isothiocynate group, which are found in crucifer-ous vegetables.

Monoterpenes

Monoterpenes are a class of phytochemicals that includes limonene, perillyl alcohol, and carvone. Monterpenes, which are a subclass of iso-prenoids, have a chemical structure that contains ten carbons. Monoter-penes are found in citrus fruits, cherries, spearmint, caraway, and dill, among other edible plants. They act as anticarcinogens because they in-duce glutathione-S-transferase activity. They also evoke a notable reduc-tion in cholesterol levels, thereby reducing the risk of heart disease.

Omega-3 Fatty Acids

Omega-3 fatty acids are essential polyunsaturated fatty acids found in abundance in the flaxseed and the leafy green purslane in the form of alpha-linolenic acid. The human body converts these plant-borne oils into the useful omega-3s eicosapentaenoic acid (EPA) and docosa-hexaenoic acid (DHA).

The importance of the omega-3 fatty acids was first gleaned from investigating the diet and rate of heart disease of Greenland Eskimos, who average a 30- to 50-gram-a-day intake of fish oil. They experience only 10 percent of the deaths from heart attack and stroke that were found in people who follow a typical Western-type diet.

Subsequent research has shown that omega-3 fatty acids are valued because of their effect on prostaglandin synthesis. Prostaglandins are hormonelike substances created in the cell for use by that cell. The prostaglandin created from omega-3 fatty acids, PG3, makes the blood cells less sticky, helps prevent or arrest tumor growth, and has the ability to enhance the immune system.

Omega-6 Fatty Acids

Omega-6 fatty acids are polyunsaturated essential fatty acids that predominate in vegetable oils derived from canola, corn, safflower, or sunflower. They are sources of linoleic acid. Omega-6 fatty acids include cis-linoleic acid, linoleic acid, and gamma-linoleic acid. They are metabolized by the body to form anti-inflammatory prostaglandins, including prostaglandin PG1, which is a weak enhancer of the immune system; although they also can be metabolized into harmful chemicals such as arachidonic acid, which synthesizes prostaglandin PG2, a strong suppressor of the immune system. Prostaglandin PG2 is found at the site of malignant cancer.

Phenols

Phenols are a class of phytochemicals that induce the phase II enzyme system. They include caffeic, chlorogenic, coumaric, ellagic, and ferulic acids, as well as quercetin and the vitamin-E containing alpha-tocopherol.

Phytosterols

Sterols are a group of alcohols that are a subgroup of steroids. Phytosterols are those sterols found in plants. They are similar in structure to cholesterol but do not have the negative effects on health that high levels of cholesterol can have, as they pass through the gastrointestinal tract almost completely unabsorbed. Since their structure is similar to that of cholesterol, they can compete with cholesterol for absorption into the bloodstream, thus lowering serum cholesterol levels. Some phytosterols also are similar in structure to the sex steroids estrogen, progesterone, and testosterone, and can thus replace these sex hormones in the body, lowering the risk for hormone-dependent cancers. Beta-sitosterol, campesterol, and stigmasterol are some of the most commonly studied of the plant sterols. Nuts, particularly peanuts, and seeds are rich sources of plant sterols. Table 1.3 shows the phytosterol content of several nuts, seeds, and seed oils.

Protease Inhibitors

Protease inhibitors are a group of phytochemicals that inhibit specific proteases in the body. A protease is an enzyme that digests proteins.

Table 1.3. Phytosterol Content of Selected Foods

Food	Amount of Phytosterol
Corn oil	1,390 mg/100 g
Corn oil, refined	952 mg/100 g
Soybean oil	327 mg/100 g
Soybean oil, refined	221 mg/100 g
Soybean oil, refined and hydrogenated	132 mg/100 g
Olive oil	232 mg/100 g
Olive oil, refined	176 mg/100 g
Sesame seeds	714 mg/100 g
Sunflower seeds	534 mg/100 g
Poppy seeds	89 mg/100 g
Peanuts	220 mg/100 g
Soybeans	161 mg/100 g
Cashews	158 mg/100 g
Almonds	143 mg/100 g
Pecans	108 mg/100 g
Kidney beans	127 mg/100 g
Broad beans	124 mg/100 g

Five protein-digesting enzymes that have specific inhibitors are trypsin, chymotrypsin, thrombin, plasmin, and elastase. Another protease inhibitor called the Bowman-Birk inhibitor differs from the others because it inactivates both chymotrypsin and trypsin. All six types are found in soybeans. Other sources are legumes, seeds, whole grains, potatoes, sweet corn, spinach, broccoli, cucumbers, Brussels sprouts, and radishes. Although it is thought that heat destroys the protease inhibitors in beans, protease inhibitors have been harvested from soybeans processed into tofu. They also have been found unchanged in chickpeas and kidney beans that have been subjected to the canning process.

In laboratory studies, protease inhibitors function as suppressors of both the initiation and the promotion of cancer. In animal studies, protease inhibitors have reduced the occurrence of tumors in animals. It appears that cancer cells produce specific proteases that act destructively and enable cancer to invade and subsequently inhabit other areas. Dietary protease inhibitors may work by flooding the protease receptor site on cells and crowding out the cancer-promoting protease, thereby keeping the cancer cell from approaching the healthy cell.

That's a brief introduction to what phytochemicals are and some of the ways they work to offer protection against disease. Certain foods have phytochemicals that appear unique in their mechanism to deflect disease. An explanation of how each phytochemical works will be explained in Chapter 3.

As we now select foods for the energy, vitamins, and minerals they offer, we may soon be finding ourselves choosing foods for their particular phytochemical content and the specific disease-fighting mechanisms they have to offer.

2

The History of Phytochemicals

 Phytochemistry is the branch of science that studies plant chemicals. It's not a new, glamorous, or exciting field—at least, not until now. The quiet world of phytochemistry has been energized by the discovery that phytochemicals found in food can prevent and fight disease. Traditionally, chemists have studied phytochemicals for the disease protection they offer plants, but they've discovered that the disease protection that phytochemicals provide plants transcends the botanical world and shields human beings from disease as well.

The term "phytochemical" debuted in the media in the spring of 1994 with a barrage of newspaper stories that culminated in a *Newsweek* cover story entitled "Better Than Vitamins: Can Phytochemicals Prevent Cancer?" That story, touting certain beneficial chemicals in plants as the disease-protective equivalent of vitamins and minerals of the twenty-first century, poised the term "phytochemical" for entry into the realm of everyday language.

In Search of Phytochemicals

Information on the disease-fighting properties of phytochemicals finally has emerged after decades of scientific detective work. Since the mid-1950s, anthropologists, botanists, statisticians, biologists, food technologists, chemists, and nutritionists have been working together to detect, isolate, analyze, and evaluate the effects of the natural food chemicals on the process of disease. Their efforts finally began to pay off in 1992 when the National Cancer Institute launched an investigation costing over $20 million to research the anticancer potential of plant foods.

The road to public recognition of a food and its phytochemicals is long and winding. The process begins by spotting how disease trends and eating habits differ culturally and geographically around the world. It then moves into the laboratory where foods are analyzed for their phytochemical content, and each phytochemical is scrutinized for its effects on the disease process with cell studies and animal studies. If these studies prove fruitful, they move into clinical human trials and can result in dietary recommendations made to the general public.

To give you an idea of the steps that are needed to bring one food and its phytochemicals to the attention of the public, consider the journey of cabbage, one of the cruciferous vegetables, and its cluster of phytochemicals as they gained acceptance for their ability to deflect disease.

A Global Effort

Cabbage first came to the attention of researchers after they observed that women living in Eastern European countries surrounding Poland and Russia were much less likely to develop breast cancer than American women. Scientists analyzed their diets, and noted, among other things, that their cabbage intake was very high, certainly higher than that of American women. When cabbage was analyzed, the phytochemicals called *indoles* emerged as one of the elements worth investigating because it seemed to alter the hormones that fueled the growth of breast cancer. Dr. H. Leon Bradlow of the Strang Cornell Cancer

Research Laboratory in New York and his team of researchers then set out to determine if indoles from cabbage could be effective in preventing breast cancer in animals.

The researchers induced breast cancer in two groups of laboratory animals and supplemented the diet of one group with indoles. The group that received the indoles developed less breast tumors, and the more indoles they were given, the fewer tumors they developed. The next phase of research involved human breast-cancer cells. The researchers found that when indoles were added to human breast-cancer cells in test tubes, they did prevent tumor growth. Then Bradlow and his team of scientists moved on to the next phase of the research. They sought to find out what would happen if the diets of humans were supplemented with indoles. They found that in the small group they supplemented, they were able to alter estrogen metabolism—estrogen is thought to fuel the growth of some breast cancers. There were no negative side effects from the ingestion of the indoles. They are now trying to determine if indoles will reduce breast-cancer rates in large groups of people.

And while the group at Strang Cornell is investigating the indoles from cabbage in New York City, another group of researchers led by Dr. Paul Talalay at Johns Hopkins Medical School in Baltimore, Maryland, is investigating another phytochemical found in cabbage, sulforaphane, for its anticancer capabilities. And at the University of Minnesota, Dr. Lee Wattenberg and his coworkers have been looking into the disease-fighting activities of the isothiocynates and dithiolethiones found in the cabbage family among the other phytochemicals they've been exploring since the 1970s. That's just a small taste of the story.

These types of investigations are simultaneously happening with other foods and their components in other parts of the world. In Italy, scientists at the University of Milan noted that the rate of prostate cancer is very low and the rate of tomato consumption is very high. At Harvard Medical School, Dr. Edward Giovannucci and his team analyzed data that were collected from 47,894 male health professionals between 1986 and 1992 in the United States. They concluded that a high intake of tomato-rich foods correlated with low rates of prostate cancer. After analyzing the components of tomatoes, they concluded that *lycopene*, a phytochemical that is a member of the carotene family, which has potent antioxidant capabilities, might offer an answer to the question "How can we prevent prostate cancer?"

The body of knowledge continues to expand. In Vidalia, Georgia, home of Vidalia onions, it was noticed that stomach-cancer rates are half the national average. Then, this information was connected to data from an ecological study done through a cooperative effort of scientists from Cornell University Medical School and the Chinese government. In northern China, where garlic production is high, scientists found the lowest national rates of stomach cancer. Onions and garlic are members of the same family, which contains the phytochemical compound *allyl sulfide*. Scientists wondered, "Could allyl sulfide have the potential to prevent stomach cancer? Is there something here worth investigating?"

The cooperative effort needed to bring this information out into the forefront is worth noting because it illustrates the positive ways in which we can operate as a global village.

A Slow Start

Although information on phytochemicals is now gaining legitimacy, the early days were less than auspicious for a number of reasons. Phytochemicals can be very elusive. One of the problems inherent in the study of phytochemicals is the variability of the phytochemical content of food. The leaf, the flower, and the stem of the same food can contain a diverse array of phytochemicals. Different varieties of the same food contain vastly different phytochemical profiles. Even two heads of broccoli of the same variety grown in different locations will vary in phytochemical content. In addition, methods and chemicals used to extract phytochemicals from foods affect the type and quantity of phytochemicals detected in food.

Bias from the established scientific research community is another reason phytochemical research has faltered. For many years, traditional researchers avoided any type of science that was related to nutrition. "Serious scientists have stayed away from the field because it gets tied up with all the supplementation people and the anti-aging crowd," said Dr. Barry Halliwell of the University of California at Davis. Dr. H. Leon Bradlow, who has been studying the link between breast cancer and hormones since 1957, expressed a similar sentiment. "Like Rodney Dangerfield, I got no respect. I was treated like a cross between a lunatic and a heretic."

Trends in medical research begin with a few visionary front-runners who forge a trail. They then pick up believers and validation along the way. Those that set the trends often pay the price of initially being branded as oddballs or mavericks.

The experiences of Dr. Kilmer McCully, a bright young Harvard medical researcher, bear examining. McCully's promising career was nearly ended thirty years ago, when he inadvertently discovered and reported that high levels of homocysteine in the blood cause severe damage to arteries and lead to heart disease. Homocysteine levels, he found, could be manipulated by adequate intake of folic acid, vitamin B_6, and vitamin B_{12}. (Folic acid is a phytonutrient that abounds in leafy green vegetables.) McCully stumbled on his discovery while investigating infants with a rare genetic defect—resulting in elevated levels of homocysteine in the blood. Their cause of death was atherosclerosis, the hardening of the arteries that is usually encountered only in the aged.

McCully hypothesized that homocysteine might damage the arteries and, like elevated cholesterol, cause problems throughout the body. He raised homocysteine levels in test animals and saw evidence of damaged arteries. He was able to prevent this from happening with adequate vitamin supplementation. His findings are now held in high regard and offer yet another plausible reason for the development of cardiovascular disease. At the time, however, his superiors at Harvard and the grant funders at the National Institutes of Health were not impressed. They were interested only in funding cholesterol-related research. Rather than receiving accolades for his work, Dr. McCully received only trouble. He fell out of favor with the scientific community, his research funding dried up, he lost his job, and he was blackballed for two years. His search for employment in his field led to dead-ends until he made moves to begin legal proceedings against his detractors. McCully eventually landed a job as a pathologist at the Providence Veteran's Administration Medical Center, and his homocysteine theory is now in the forefront of the research on heart disease prevention.

Gaining Momentum

Although the field of phytochemical research is slowly gaining esteem and has been deemed worthy of funding by the National Institutes of Health, phytochemicals are not new in government circles. The United States Department of Agriculture has the Phytochemeco database. This catalogue of all the phytochemicals that have been isolated from foods is a work in progress that has been painstakingly developed by botanist James Duke over twenty years.

Raising money for the funding of phytochemical studies is still a problem that was expressed at an international conference titled "Dietary Phytochemicals in Cancer Prevention and Treatment," which took place in Washington, D.C., in late August of 1995. Excited researchers from all over the world met and took their turns at the podium to share findings about foods, their phytochemicals, and the methods with which they fight disease. At an after-hours session, scientists took the time to brainstorm ways of raising money for furthering their research goals. Research findings and ideas for future studies were plentiful, but it was agreed that funds for conducting research were less than abundant. It is hoped that, as phytochemical-rich foods' reputation for fighting disease grows, phytochemical studies will command larger percentages of the health-care research dollar.

CHEMOPREVENTION — WHERE HISTORY MEETS THE FUTURE

The discovery of the ability of phytochemicals to stymie the disease process led to the term "chemoprevention," which was coined in the mid-1970s by Michael B. Sporn, an innovator in cancer prevention research, to characterize a new approach to preventing disease with the use of plant food or its components. In the early 1980s, the National Cancer Institute Chemoprevention Program of the Division of Cancer

Prevention and Control was created to investigate the scientific value of the many food components identified as chemopreventive. In 1997, the Division of Cancer Prevention and Control was disbanded, and two new separate divisions were established—the Division of Cancer Prevention and the Division of Cancer Control and Population Sciences. The concept of chemoprevention leads us into a new arena in disease prevention and raises many new questions. What are the optimal levels for phytochemical intake? Is there any preferred method of achieving optimal levels? Is there any value to foods being engineered to have exceptional amounts of phytochemicals?

Optimal Intakes of Phytochemicals for Chemoprevention

Currently, there are no established optimal levels for phytochemical intake. The USDA recommends that the majority of one's diet be composed of those foods on the lower tiers of the Food Guide Pyramid—fruits, vegetables, and whole grains. Including five servings of fruits and vegetables daily in our diets ensures that we obtain an adequate intake of health-providing phytochemicals. We should also consider frequently selecting our protein from plant, nut, and legume sources, since they come with a bonus in the form of phytochemicals.

Research indicates that recommendations for optimal phytochemical intake might vary based on personal health status. When determining the optimal intake needed for micronutrients, it appears that optimal intake is related to baseline serum levels of key nutrients—that is, the amount you start out with before supplementation. The phytochemical intake needed to maintain health might be substantially different from the amount needed in the presence of active disease.

The research necessary to determine guidelines for optimal intake of phytochemicals to achieve chemoprevention is inconclusive at this time. However, common sense dictates that it would be wise to err on the side of more rather than less phytochemically rich foods to work toward a chemopreventive diet.

Obtaining Phytonutrients: Diet Versus Supplementation

Phytochemical supplements are taking their place on the shelves of drug and natural food stores next to vitamins and minerals. However, supplements may not be as useful in maintaining optimal health as is a phytochemical-rich diet. Studies designed to measure the effects of supplementation with the antioxidant beta-carotene on the prevention of both lung and colorectal cancer have been disappointing for supplement advocates and have demonstrated the superiority of fruits and vegetables as a method of disease prevention. Although high serum levels of beta-carotene and increased fruit and vegetable intake are markers of decreased risk of lung and colon cancers, supplementation with beta-carotene did not decrease cancer in clinical trials designed to test its effectiveness. Preliminary research indicates that increased intake of fruits and vegetables is the preferred method of achieving chemopreventive doses of phytochemicals.

Another reason to choose food over supplements when seeking phytochemicals is that the study of phytochemicals is an emerging science. In addition to the phytochemicals that scientists are already familiar with, there are bound to be many as yet undiscovered compounds in vegetable foods that amplify health. If they have not yet been discovered, they cannot be included in supplements. Furthermore, phytochemicals probably work in conjunction with other nutrients found in plants, such as vitamins and minerals. It is probably best to consume phytochemicals, as well as vitamins and minerals, in the form that nature presents them to us. To best achieve chemopreventive levels of phytochemicals, a daily intake of at least five fruits and vegetables as part of a varied diet is the preferred method.

Engineered Foods

Foods that are fortified or genetically engineered are alternate methods of adding chemopreventive phytochemicals to the diet. Such foods are referred to as either functional foods or designer foods. Functional foods and designer foods are foods that are supplemented with ingredients naturally rich in disease-preventing substances. This may involve genetic engineering of food. Vitamin-C enriched oranges, high-phytochemical broccoflower (a combination of broccoli and cauliflower), and fiber-enriched baked goods have already begun to appear in the market. The benefit that these foods provide is that the consumer will be meeting nutrient needs while at the same time consuming extra phytochemicals.

THE FUTURE OF PHYTOCHEMICALS

It is as if a dam burst and let flow a river of new information that will enable us to take more control of our own health. And the timing could not be better. The high cost of health care is putting a strain on personal budgets and government funds. This new information about phytochemicals can further guide us in our food choices to take control of our health.

Making Phytochemical Information User Friendly

We will need concise and accessible information to make phytochemicals user friendly and part of our national consciousness. In time, phytochemical information needs to be moved into its rightful place in the existing database that is managed by the United States Department of Agriculture called the Nutrient Database for Standard Reference. There, it will take its place next to the vitamins and minerals and calories in foods, providing more information that can be accessed for diet planning.

Drugs That Act Like Foods

Phytochemicals might have their greatest impact as inspirations for the creation of new pharmaceuticals. Drugs that imitate the mechanisms of phytochemicals are now being designed. Many of the new cancer drugs that are being developed seek to do what phytochemicals from foods already accomplish. Drugs are being created to interfere with the creation of new blood vessels so that tumors cannot get the nutrients they need to develop a blood supply and spread throughout the body. This is how genistein, which abounds in soy foods, works. The drug tamoxifen acts as an anti-estrogen, however, as do the isoflavone phytochemicals and lignans. Drugs are being developed that inhibit the activation of tyrosine kinase and prevent growth signals from reaching a tumor cell; the isoflavone genistein does that, too.

While medicine might be taking its inspiration from nature, drugs never seem to offer a benefit without a negative side effect. By using plant food as medicine, you get the benefits of the phytochemicals without the undesirable side effects.

If I were writing a movie script, I could not set the scene more dramatically—as the century closes, we enter an exciting new frontier in the annals of nutrition. Are we reaching an era where it is appropriate to recommend one food over another for its phytochemical content? Should we be more specific when we recommend five fruits and vegetables a day? Should we indicate which plant groups to choose from to get optimal disease protection? This has not yet been decided. We have a lot more to learn, but it's certainly beginning to appear that increased plant food consumption might offer one safe, cost-effective method of lowering the high cost of health care.

Phytochemicals from A to Z

3

As you already know from reading the previous chapters, science has identified hundreds of phytochemicals. Some of these phytochemicals distinguish themselves because they exert more powerful disease-fighting mechanisms than others do. This chapter contains a roll call of the most powerful biologically active phytochemicals that appear in foods.

In each entry, you will find an explanation of how the phytochemical works and what foods it is found in, along with a pronunciation key to help facilitate a discussion of the phytochemicals. In some instances, when more than one correct pronunciation exists, I have provided the most commonly used pronunciation. From each passage, you will gain an explicit understanding of the ways that each phytochemical affects your health.

AJOENE *(a-HO-een).* Ajoene is a phytochemical found in garlic that makes blood platelets less sticky and inhibits blood-clot formation. It is thought to be at least as potent as aspirin in its ability to deter the aggregation of blood platelets. It has not been found in dehydrated garlic powder or in garlic pills, oils, or extracts. Researchers believe that the process of steam distillation used in the preparation of garlic supplements destroys ajoene. One or two cloves of raw or slightly cooked garlic will probably provide a disease-preventive dose.

ALLICIN *(AL-li-sin).* Allicin is found in garlic and is responsible for its odor. It is released from the garlic upon bruising or cutting into it. The more cuts made in the garlic, the more allicin is released. It may lower cholesterol, blood pressure, and the risk of cancer. Allicin, which is related to the phytochemical diallyl sulfide, is detected in fresh garlic, dehydrated garlic powder, and some garlic supplements. Table 3.1 indicates the quantity of allicin found in a variety of sources.

ALPHA-LINOLENIC *(AL-fuh lin-o-LEN-ick)* **ACID.** Alpha-linolenic acid is an omega-3 fatty acid found in soy, flaxseed, and rapeseed oil, as well as in some leafy green vegetables. The human body converts alpha-linolenic acid into eicosapentaenoic acid (EPA) and, more slowly, into docosahexaenoic acid (DHA), the valuable essential oils found in

Table 3.1. Levels of Allicin Detected in Garlic Supplements

Item	Quantity	Levels of Allicin
Fresh garlic	One clove	5,000 mcg
Garlic powder (Schilling)	⅓ tsp	5,600 mcg
KAL Beyond Garlic	1 pill	3,500 mcg
Garlaction	1 pill	800 mcg
Garlicin	1 pill	2,500 mcg
Life Garlic	1 pill	300 mcg
Kwai	1 pill	700 mcg
Solaray Garlicare	1 pill	4,000 mcg

fish, as needed. Alpha-linolenic acid is related to EPA and DHA in much the same way that beta-carotene is related to vitamin A—it is a precursor.

ALPHA-TOCOPHEROL *(AL-fuh to-KO-fer-awl)*. Alpha-tocopherol is the form that vitamin E takes in plants. A major function of vitamin E is its role as an antioxidant. Vitamin E protects polyunsaturated fatty acids in cell membranes from being attacked by free radicals. It also inhibits the formation of nitrosamines. The Recommended Dietary Allowance of vitamin E for adult men and women is approximately 30 IU daily. Larger doses are used therapeutically to prevent the oxidative damage that is believed to lead to heart disease. Current research indicates that 50 IU of alpha-tocopherol a day may cut the risk of prostate cancer; 100 IU may reduce the risk of heart disease; and 200 to 400 IU may boost the immune system of the elderly. Vitamin E is found in the plant world in whole grains, nuts, seeds, wheat germ, asparagus, and lettuce.

ANETHOFURAN *(AN-eh-tho-FYOOR-an)*. Anethofuran is a phytochemical found in the dill weed plant. It induces the anticancer detoxifying enzyme glutathione-S-transferase.

ANETHOLE *(AN-eh-thole)*. Anethole is a phytochemical found in the peppermint plant. It acts as a carminative to expel gas from the bowels and as a digestive aid because it stimulates activity in the stomach and small intestines. It also increases the flow of breast milk.

ANTHOCYANINS *(AN-tho-SIE-uh-nins)*. Anthocyanins are the reddish-blue pigments found in cherries, cranberries, raspberries, blueberries, grapes, red currants, and red cabbage. There are over 150 different anthocyanins in the plant world. They inhibit cholesterol synthesis by limiting the production of HMG-COA reductase, a precursor to cholesterol. This may make anthocyanins protective against both cancer and heart disease.

ASCORBIC *(as-COR-bik)* **ACID.** Ascorbic acid is the plant form of vitamin C. It is found in a variety of fruits and vegetables, most notably citrus fruits and their juices, broccoli, green pepper, and tomatoes. It is sensitive to heat and can be destroyed by cooking. In addition to its role as an antioxidant, vitamin C also works in the stomach to bind with nitrates and prevent the formation of carcinogenic nitrosamines. It is needed for formation of collagen, which is an integral part of connective tissue structure. The majority of population studies—thirty-three out of forty-six—showed an inverse relationship between vitamin C intake and cancer risk, meaning the more vitamin C present, the lower the cancer risk. A high intake of vitamin C appears to decrease cancer risk by 50 percent. The Recommended Dietary Allowance of vitamin C is 60 milligrams; however, the optimal dose probably resides between 60 and 1,000 milligrams, depending upon one's health status. Research shows that doses that exceed 2,000 to 3,000 milligrams may actually impede immunity.

ASPARAGUS CRUDE SAPONINS *(SAY-po-ninz)*. Asparagus crude saponins (ACS), found in the edible shoots of the asparagus plant, inhibited the growth of human leukemia cells in a cell study done at Rutgers University. It is thought that asparagus crude saponins act on leukemia cells by decreasing the rate of cell reproduction and of DNA synthesis. The ACS worked on the human leukemia cells in a dose- and time-dependent manner, which means the rate of inhibition of the leukemia cells depended on how much asparagus crude saponin was used and how long the leukemia cells were exposed to the phytochemical.

BENZYL ISOTHIOCYNATE *(BEN-zil IGH-so-THIGh-oh-SIGH-nate)*. Benzyl isothiocynate has the distinction of having both blocking and suppressing actions against cancer. As a blocking agent it helps prevent cancer before it is established, and as a suppressing agent it works to inhibit the expression of cancer in its earliest stages.

It is believed that a tumor forms because its DNA gets an incorrect message. Benzyl isothiocynate works as a suppressor of a tumor by blocking this message. Consider this example: You turn on the radio, and all you get is static. You find that if you stand in a certain place near the radio, the sound clears—you suppress the static. When you move, the static returns. That is how a suppressing agent works. It has to be present constantly to suppress the tumor. So, it follows that you would need a steady supply of benzyl isothiocynate if you want to suppress tumor growth. Benzyl isothiocynate is present in the family of cruciferous vegetables, including Brussels sprouts, cabbage, kale, cauliflower, broccoli, collard greens, kohlrabi, rutabaga, turnips, arugula, and watercress. A daily serving of at least one of these vegetables could offer a chemopreventive dose.

BETA-CAROTENE (*BAY-tuh CAR-uh-teen*). Beta-carotene is a yellow-orange pigment in some fruits and vegetables. It is a member of the carotenoid family of phytochemicals. Beta-carotene is converted into vitamin A by the liver and fulfills all of the biological tasks of vitamin A. In its role as an antioxidant, beta-carotene helps to stabilize unstable free-radical molecules. By offering itself as a sacrifice, it prevents free radicals from damaging cells. To some extent, beta-carotene is found in all green vegetables, but its yellow-orange pigment is masked by chlorophyll. It is found abundantly in sweet potatoes, carrots, spinach, and butternut and acorn squash. Fruits that are rich sources of beta-carotene are cantaloupe, mango, papaya, and apricots.

The Recommended Dietary Allowance for retinol equivalents (carotenes) is 800 to 1,000 micrograms. Try to consume at least this much daily. A 3.5-ounce serving of sweet potato with the skin on contains twice that amount. Excessive beta-carotene consumption can result in hypercarotenemia, a harmless condition in which the skin turns an orangish color due to the liver's inability to process all of the beta-carotene into vitamin A. Excess carotene is stored in the skin and lends an orange pigment to flesh that is initially visible in the palms of the hands.

BETA-GLUCAN (*BAY-tuh GLOO-kan*). Beta-glucan is the main soluble fiber portion of oat bran. (See "Fiber" on page 44.)

BETA-SITOSTEROL (*BAY-tuh SIGH-to-STER-awl*). Beta-sitosterol is found in nuts, seeds, and saw palmetto and, to a lesser extent, in almost all plants. Beta-sitosterol supplementation in animal studies resulted in decreased formation of chemically induced tumors of the colon. In addition, beta-sitosterol can block cholesterol absorption from the diet or increase cholesterol excretion from the body. One study found that one gram (1,000 milligrams) of beta-sitosterol reduced the absorption of cholesterol from a meal containing 500 milligrams of cholesterol by 42 percent. Beta-sitosterol appears to prevent the conversion of testosterone into dihydrotestosterone. A buildup of dihydrotestosterone plays a major role in the development of benign prostatic hyperplasia, the inflammatory nonmalignant enlargement of the prostate gland that leads to many urinary problems for the majority of men over fifty years old.

A 1995 clinical study in Germany performed on 200 men with benign hyperplasia of the prostate demonstrated that those supplemented with the phytosterols beta-sitosterol, campesterol, and stigmasterol showed significant improvement in symptoms and urinary flow over those in the control group who were given a placebo—an inert substance. The fruit of the saw palmetto tree, which is very rich in the phytosterols, is a well-known herbal remedy for the symptoms of benign hyperplasia of the prostate.

BOWMAN-BIRK *(BOH-men-BERK)* **INHIBITOR.** Bowman-Birk inhibitor (BBI) is a protease inhibitor that is a potent anticarcinogen. A protease is a protein-digesting enzyme. BBI is unique because it inactivates the proteases chymotrypsin and trypsin, whereas most protease inhibitors suppress only one protease. It is found in soybeans and is thought to be inactivated by heat. The addition of 0.5-percent Bowman-Birk inhibitor to the diet of a particular breed of mice called Min mice, who are genetically predisposed to developing cancerous tumors of the small and large intestines, resulted in a 40-percent decrease in tumors when contrasted with the control group.

BROMELAIN *(BRO-muh-lane)*. Bromelain is a protein-digesting enzyme in pineapples that has been recognized since 1876. It has been used in therapeutic doses since 1957. In clinical trials, bromelain has demonstrated the ability to decrease the viscosity of mucus in 124 patients hospitalized with chronic bronchitis. It has been used successfully as a digestive enzyme following pancreatic surgery. It has demonstrated therapeutic effects in the treatment of inflammation and soft tissue injuries, particularly when administered prior to injury, as evidenced by a clinical trial of 74 boxers and 55 presurgical patients. Bromelain also demonstrated the ability to reduce blood clotting in 85 percent of people when tested on a group of 20 with a history of stroke, heart attack, or high platelet-aggregation values.

CAFFEIC *(ka-FAY-ick)* **ACID.** Caffeic acid is a phenolic phytochemical that is widely distributed in plants. Caffeic acid is listed as an anti-HIV phytochemical in the United States Department of Agriculture's database on phytochemicals. With ferulic acid, another common phytochemical, caffeic acid has been shown to decrease both lung and skin tumors in animal experiments. Caffeic and ferulic acids induce the body's own ability to detoxify harmful substances. In addition, they trap the potential cancer-causing nitrates and deactivate them. They are found in large amounts in apples, potatoes, and lettuce, and to a lesser extent in strawberries and Brussels sprouts.

CALCIUM *(KAL-see-um).* Though calcium is most known to be found in milk, this mineral is abundant in plants as well and is found in leafy greens and legumes. It is used by the body to build bones and teeth and also plays a critical role in muscle action and thereby helps to maintain the heartbeat. Calcium must be present for muscles to work and for the nervous system to function and transmit impulses. If calcium is not supplied by the diet, the body will extract calcium from the skeletal system for use in maintaining the nervous system. Constant use of calcium by the body without dietary replenishment can lead to osteoporosis later in life. Tofu is often enriched with calcium, making such varieties good sources of the mineral. It was once believed that oxalates and phytates, which are also found in plants, impeded the availability of plant-based calcium to the body. More recent animal studies, however, have shown no difference in the absorption of calcium from tofu than from dairy sources. The Recommended Dietary Allowance (RDA) of calcium is 1,300 milligrams for both males and females nine to eighteen years old; 1,000 milligrams for adults nineteen to fifty; and 1,200 milligrams for adults fifty-one and over. This amount should be adequate for maintaining optimal health. Table 3.2 depicts how vegetable sources of calcium compare to milk.

Table 3.2. Availability of Calcium from Dairy and Plant Sources

Food	Quantity	Calcium Content	Calcium Available for Use
Milk	8 ounces	300 mg	96.3 mg
Tofu	4 ounces	258 mg	80 mg
Kale	½ cup	47 mg	27 mg
Broccoli	½ cup	35 mg	18.4 mg
Pinto beans	½ cup	45 mg	17 mg
Spinach	½ cup	122 mg	6.2 mg

CAMPESTEROL *(KAM-peh-STER-awl).* Campesterol is a phytosterol that might be useful in treating benign hyperplasia of the prostate gland. It is found in beans and oils.

CAPSAICIN *(kap-SAY-sin).* Capsaicin is a phytochemical isolated from red peppers that acts as an anti-inflammatory and is used topically for relief from arthritis pain. It also suppresses cholesterol formation in the liver.

CARNOSOL *(KAR-nuh-sawl).* Carnosol is found in the herb rosemary. It has demonstrated anticancer activity in animal studies. When mice were exposed to a known carcinogen that causes breast cancer, carnosol increased the production of an enzyme that protected the cellular DNA from being damaged. Carnosol also has the ability to destroy candida yeast.

CARVACROL *(KAR-vuh-krawl).* Carvacrol is a phytochemical found in the herbs bergamot, thyme, wild savory, and rosemary. In test tube studies, it has shown the ability to prevent the breakdown of acetylcholine, a neurotransmitter involved in the processes of learning and memory. Carvacrol also has anticandida activity.

CARVEOL *(KAR-vee-awl).* Carveol is a monoterpene. It is also one of the smaller isoprenoid phytochemicals, consisting of two isoprene units.

It is present in dill and caraway seeds. It induces the detoxifying enzyme glutathione-S-transferase and inhibits HMG-COA reductase activity, which may make it beneficial in protecting against cancer and heart disease.

CHLOROGENIC *(KLOR-o-JEN-ick)* **ACID.** Chlorogenic acid is a phenolic phytochemical that acts as blocking agent against cancer. It is found at highest levels in freshly harvested fruits and vegetables. This phytochemical traps nitrates, inhibiting them from forming potentially carcinogenic nitrosamines. It is listed as an anti-HIV phytochemical in the United States Department of Agriculture's database on phytochemicals. Chlorogenic acid is found in almost all fruits and vegetables.

CHLOROPHYLL *(KLOR-uh-fil).* Chlorophyll, the green pigment of leaves and plants, fights bedsores and bad breath and prevents cancer and excessive bleeding, according to the USDA phytochemical database. It is also known to work as a deodorant. Maté tea, grown in South America, is one of the richest known sources of chlorophyll.

CITRONELLOL *(sit-run-EL-awl).* Citronellol is found in corn leaves, ginger root, sweet basil, and winter savory. It has candidacide and antibacterial properties.

COUMARINS *(COO-mer-inz).* Coumarins induce the anticancer detoxifying enzyme glutathione-S-transferase (GST) in the livers and small intestines of mice. They are thought to block carcinogens and have inhibited tumors in animal experiments. Coumarins are widely distributed in vegetables and citrus fruits.

CURCUMIN *(ker-KYOO-min).* Curcumin is the principal active compound and the major yellow coloring in the spice turmeric, a component of curry powder. It offers a protective effect against cancer because it has the potential to block the spread of a tumor, a process known as metastasis. This phenolic phytochemical has strong antioxidant activities. It also inhibits the formation of carcinogenic nitrate compounds. In a study designed to test the power of curcumin to guard against cancer, rats were treated with a known colon carcinogen. The group of rats treated with curcumin developed 34-percent fewer cancers. The tumors that did develop in the curcumin-treated rats were smaller and less invasive than the tumors in the control group, which did not receive curcumin.

Curcumin also has anti-inflammatory properties. "Curcumin apparently shuts off certain transcription factors—switches that turn on the machinery of the cell that are absolutely critical for inflammation," said Bharat B. Aggarwal, Ph.D., chief of the cytokine research section at the University of Texas M.D. Anderson Cancer Center in Houston. Other research studies suggest that curcumin can help prevent cataracts and support its traditional use as an antiwrinkle preparation.

DAIDZEIN (*DAID-zeen*). Daidzein is an isoflavone that is found principally in legumes. It has potential as an anticancer agent and has been investigated as a possible treatment for alcoholism.

DIALLYL SULFIDE (*die-AL-lil SUL-fide*). Diallyl sulfide (DAS), which is related to the phytochemical allicin, increases glutathione-S-transferase (GST) activity in the stomach. It is found in onions, garlic, leeks, Chinese chives, and shallots.

DITHIOLETHIONE (*die-THIGH-ol-THIGH-own*). Dithiolethione is a phytochemical that induces the phase II anticancer enzyme glutathione-S-transferase (GST), which stimulates the antioxidant glutathione. Dithiolethione is present in the family of cruciferous vegetables—Brussels sprouts, cabbage, kale, cauliflower, broccoli, collard greens, kohlrabi, rutabaga, turnips, arugula, and watercress. In animal studies, it acts as a blocking agent against cancer in the lungs, liver, midsection of the small intestine, and the kidney. When animal tumors were induced by administration of aflatoxin, a cancer-causing agent found in food, those animals fed dithiolethione demonstrated between 40- and 80-percent less pretumor activity. Like many other carcinogens, aflatoxin needs to be activated to be harmful. Dithiolethione blocks the activation of aflatoxin. When dithiolethione is administered, there is less binding of aflatoxin to the DNA. It is the binding of the carcinogen, in this case aflatoxin, to the DNA in the cell that presumably causes the initial damage responsible for the altered cell growth seen in cancer. In large segments of the world, much of the food supply is contaminated with aflatoxin, and a major cause of death is liver cancer. Dithiolethione has the ability to block the activation of aflatoxin in animals.

ELLAGIC (*EL-luh-jik*) **ACID.** Ellagic acid is a phenolic phytochemical that blocks the initiation stage of cancer. It is found in grapes; berries, including strawberries, raspberries, blackberries, and cranberries; and nuts.

EPIGALLOCATECHIN-3-GALLATE (*EP-ee-GAL-oh-KAT-e-kin THREE GAL-ate*). Epigallocatechin-3-gallate (EGCG) is a polyphenol found in green tea. Green tea is commonly consumed in China and Japan in quantities as high as ten cups a day. In the laboratory, green tea consumed at the rate of four or more cups a day was experimentally shown to decrease tumor initiation, decrease tumor progression, and cause the regression of established tumors of the skin. It is also a significant cholesterol-lowering agent. These actions may be due to the presence of EGCG.

It is believed that EGCG has the ability to inhibit the action of the enzyme urokinase, which enables cancer cells to invade other cells and metastasize. In animal models, green tea was fed to or used topically on mice whose skin cancer was induced by exposure to ultraviolet radiation B. Continual oral feedings of green tea was shown to significantly decrease tumor induction. Topical exposure of mice to green tea was not as effective as the ingestion of the tea. The scientists concluded that green tea might reduce the induction of skin cancer in humans from ultraviolet radiation.

Green tea also has offered protection in animal models against lung cancer and colon cancer at all stages of cancer. The American Institute for Cancer Research has stated that there is convincing evidence that green tea reduces the risk of stomach cancer, perhaps due to EGCG.

ERITADENINE (*e-RIT-uh-de-neen*). Eritadenine is a phytochemical isolated from shiitake mushrooms. In a study of Japanese men, participants who ate four ounces of fresh shiitake mushrooms or two ounces of dried shiitake mushrooms had a 10-percent drop in cholesterol within one week. Animal studies corroborate these findings. In a study done in Japan, eritadenine lowered cholesterol in rats that were fed various types of oils. Regardless of the fat source, eritadenine was able to lower cholesterol.

EUGENOL *(yoo-JEN-awl)*. Eugenol has been found in abundance in the clove flower. It is also present in allspice and the ginger root. According to the USDA phytochemical and ethnobotanical database, it has antiseptic, anticoagulant, and candidacide actions.

FENCHON *(FEN-chahn)*. Fenchon is a phytochemical isolated from the herb rosemary. It is documented as having potential anti-Alzheimer's action; as evidenced in test tubes, it has the ability to prevent the breakdown of acetylcholine, a neurotransmitter involved in the processes of learning and memory.

FERRULIC *(fer-ROO-lick)* **ACID.** Ferulic acid is widely distributed throughout the plant world. With caffeic acid, this phytochemical has been shown to decrease both lung and skin tumors in animal experiments.

FIBER *(FIGH-ber)*. Fiber found in plant foods is a phytochemical. Dietary fiber is found in vegetables, fruits, legumes, nuts, seeds, and grains.

The type of fiber found in whole grains is mostly *insoluble,* which means that it does not break down in water. It is also indigestible, so it adds bulk to the digestive contents, speeding up the movement of food through the digestive tract. It provides relief from constipation and diverticulosis and may help to reduce the risk of colon cancer. The role that insoluble fiber plays in disease prevention is well documented.

Soluble fiber is found in fruits and vegetables, beans, legumes, seeds, oats—particularly the bran portion of unrefined oats—and barley. Soluble fiber forms a gel in the intestines. This gel traps cholesterol and bile acids and increases their excretion. In this way, soluble fiber plays an important role in the regulation and prevention of cardiovascular disease. The recommended daily intake of fiber is 25 to 35 grams for healthy adults.

FLAVONOIDS *(FLAY-vuh-noydz)*. Flavonoids are a large family of phenolic phytochemicals that can be metabolized by the human body. There are about 800 different flavonoids found in the plant world.

Some work synergistically with the vitamin C found in citrus fruit to build capillary walls. This makes some flavonoids critically important in healing and in the prevention of bruising. Other flavonoids are anti-inflammatory, antihepatoxic (working against liver toxins), antitumor-forming, antimicrobial, antiviral, antioxidant, anti-allergenic, anti-ulcer, and analgesic. They have extensive biological properties that promote health. Some flavonoids induce the cytochrome p450 system (see page 9), while others inhibit it. Flavonoids are widely distributed in plant foods.

FOLIC *(FAH-lick)* **ACID.** Folic acid is a B vitamin whose name is derived from the word "foliage," which is a good indication of where it's found in food. Good sources of folic acid are spinach, asparagus, and turnip greens, as well as legumes.

Folic acid reduces homocysteine levels in the blood. High homocysteine levels are a risk factor for cardiovascular disease. Adequate folic acid intake is needed for women of childbearing age to prevent the birth of babies with neural tubal birth defects. The administration of folic acid has been known to reverse the often precancerous condition cellular dysplasia, which can occur in the cervix and the lungs. The current recommended dosage of folic acid is 400 micrograms daily for the maintenance of good health. The upper tolerable level of folic acid for adults is 1,000 micrograms per day.

FRUCTOOLIGOSACCHARIDES *(FROOK-to-o-LIG-o-SAK-a-rides).* Fructooligosaccharides (FOS) are indigestible but fermentable carbohydrates that occur naturally in common foods such as onions, bananas, tomatoes, barley, garlic, and wheat. They are found most abundantly in the Jerusalem artichoke plant. They pass through the small intestine undigested and are fermented in the colon by helpful *bifidobacteria* into short-chain fatty acids. These short-chain fatty acids create an environment in the colon that does not support the growth of harmful bacteria—giving the beneficial bacteria an edge. Therefore, FOS-containing foods may be helpful to people in whom the balance of good and potentially bad bacteria has been disrupted, such as in people taking antibiotics or undergoing chemotherapy.

FOS also can play a role in the management of diabetes. Some studies have shown that fructooligosaccharides, when used in place of another carbohydrate, will produce less of an increase in blood glucose and insulin levels as compared with other carbohydrates. FOS supplements have been tested in a variety of clinical trials and have been well tolerated when dosage does not exceed 25 grams per day. Table 3.3 indicates the amount of FOS in various plant foods.

FURANOCOUMARINS (*foo-RAN-oh-COO-mer-inz*). Furanocoumarins are phytochemicals abundant in grapefruit but not found in other citrus fruits. When a person drinks the juice, these furanocoumarins bind to a set of enzymes in the lining of the intestines called CYP 3A4 en-

Table 3.3. Foods Containing Fructooligosaccharides (FOS)

Food	Amount of FOS
Apple, red delicious	0.1 mg/g
Artichoke, globe	2.4 mg/g
Artichoke, Jerusalem	58.4 mg/g
Banana, ripe	2.0 mg/g
Blackberries	0.2 mg/g
Carrot	0.3 mg/g
Garlic	3.9 mg/g
Leek	0.9 mg/g
Onion, yellow	2.6 mg/g
Onion powder	45.0 mg/g
Orange, navel	0.3 mg/g
Peach	0.4 mg/g
Pear, d'Anjou	0.2 mg/g
Peas, snap	1.1 mg/g
Potato, sweet	0.2 mg/g
Shallot	8.5 mg/g
Watermelon	0.2 mg/g

zymes. These enzymes break down certain drugs, eventually stopping the drugs' actions. Ordinarily, hindering these enzymes doesn't cause any problems, unless a person drinks grapefruit juice to swallow a medication that is usually broken down by CYP 3A4 enzymes before being absorbed into the bloodstream. The enzymes are then not available to break down the drug, so a more active drug remains in the intestines and may be absorbed into the bloodstream over a longer period of time. The end result is that a person receives a higher dose of the medication. Drugs affected by grapefruit juice are Halcion, Versed, Plendil, Procardia, Seldane, Sandimmune, Adalat, Invirase, Tegretol, and Mevacor.

GENISTEIN *(JEN-i-steen)*. Genistein is an isoflavone found in legumes. It is very well absorbed by the human digestive tract. Among the isoflavones, genistein has the highest binding affinity for estrogen receptors, as well as some estrogenic activity, and thus it is considered a phytoestrogen. Genistein is the ingredient thought to give soy foods their ability to minimize the irritating symptoms of menopause. It also is being investigated for its ability to retard osteoporosis. Its use as an inhibitor of hormone-dependent cancers is controversial because of its mild estrogenic activity. Genistein also acts specifically as an inhibitor of the enzyme tyrosine kinase, which is associated with the sending of signals from cellular growth factor receptors that are found in abundance in cancerous cells. Tyrosine kinase is active in hormone-independent cancers as well as hormone-dependent cancers. Tyrosine kinase also encourages the aggregation of blood platelets, which leads to blockages in the cardiovascular system. This suggests that the genistein found in legumes might be useful in inhibiting both cancer and cardiovascular disease.

GERANIOL *(jer-AY-nee-awl)*. Geraniol is an isoprenoid found in grape leaves, wild bergamot (which is used to flavor Earl Grey tea), carrots, thyme, cinnamon, rosemary, and ginger. It is useful in blocking and suppressing both cancer and cardiovascular disease. It also has the ability to destroy the yeast candida.

GINGEROLE (*JIN-jer-ole*). Gingerole is a phytochemical that is found in gingerroot. It is listed in the United States Department of Agriculture's phytochemical database as an anti-emetic, which means that it inhibits nausea and vomiting. Gingerole is used in Europe for treating morning sickness from pregnancy and motion sickness. It also acts as an antitussive to treat coughs and the congestion associated with colds and flu.

GLUCARATES (*GLOO-ker-ates*). Glucarates are phytochemicals that are believed to have the ability to block the DNA damage that leads to breast cancer. Glucarates are found in the white membrane, or the albedo, of the citrus fruit and also are being studied for their potential to reduce the symptoms of premenstrual syndrome.

GLYCYRRHIZA (*glis-er-RIZE-a*). Glycyrrhiza is the phytochemical found in the licorice plant. Licorice is one of the foods that the National Cancer Institute is studying for its anticancer properties. It is one of the few natural sweeteners that does not increase thirst. In addition, it increases the body's ability to retain water.

INDOLE-3-CARBINOL (*IN-dole THREE CAR-bin-awl*). Indole-3-carbinol (I3C) is formed when broccoli or other cruciferous vegetables are chewed. The action of chewing releases the enzyme myrosinase from one compartment in the vegetable cell, whereupon it is mixed with another enzyme (glucobrassicin); together they form the active phytochemical indole-3-carbinol.

I3C is a phytochemical that fights cancer in a variety of ways. It acts as a blocking agent against cancer-causing substances by inducing the activity of the phase II enzyme glutathione-S-transferase, but at the same time it stimulates the mixed-function oxidase system. It also helps to guide estrogen metabolism and steers estrogen production toward a more benign, less toxic estrogen that does not promote the growth of estrogen-dependent cancers.

In human studies, I3C has shown specific antigrowth effects in human breast cancer cells. When I3C is administered with or prior to a known cancer-causing agent, it offers a chemoprotective effect. In several studies, mice and rats treated with I3C before exposure to a known carcinogenic agent showed a decreased incidence of mammary tumors compared with those not treated with I3C. Tumors that did develop were smaller and less virulent. It is notable that in the cabbage-eating countries of Eastern Europe that surround the easternmost border of Russia, fewer cases of breast cancer are reported. Indole-3-carbinol is found in the family of cruciferous vegetables: Brussels sprouts, cabbage, kale, cauliflower, broccoli, collard greens, kohlrabi, rutabaga, turnips, arugula, and watercress. There is great variation in the amount of I3C among different varieties of the same vegetable. Deviations appear to stem chiefly from growing conditions, plant genetics, and age at the time of harvest.

All About Indole-3-Carbinol and Estrogen

By now, you are probably aware that there are two types of cholesterol: the bad, artery-clogging LDL and the good, artery-cleaning HDL. Now scientists are saying we should think of estrogen, particularly its metabolites, in a similar dual way. There's a good estrogen metabolite, C-2, and there's a less-than-good estrogen metabolite, C-16. The I3C formed from cruciferous vegetables favors the production of C-2 estrogen as opposed to C-16 estrogen.

Estrogen is produced chiefly in the ovaries. It travels throughout the bloodstream, latching on to estrogen receptor sites that are located primarily in the female reproductive system. Once linked up, estrogen goes to work helping to ensure reproductive functioning. Finally, when its task is finished, the estrogen is degraded into its metabolites C-2 or C-16. This is where I3C does its job. I3C helps guide the breakdown of estrogen metabolites and favors the production of the more benign C-2 estrogen.

The C-16 estrogen metabolite is associated with malignant breast tumors because it is often found in high concentrations at the site of the tumor. C-16 estrogen is stimulated by excessive alcohol consumption and exposure to environmental toxins. It is

(continued on page 50)

(continued from page 49)

found in higher concentrations in women who have diets that are high in fat and have an increased percentage of body fat.

The C-2 estrogen metabolite, on the other hand, is a safer, less toxic pathway for estrogen to take. It is associated with low-fat diets, low body fat, and increased aerobic exercise. All of these factors are inversely related to hormone-related cancers, meaning the more these factors are present, the fewer hormone-dependent cancers are present. The C-2 estrogen is found in increased concentration in the urine of women who are marathon runners.

It has been demonstrated that production of C-2 estrogen can be induced by increasing one's intake of I3C. When I3C was given to both men and women in the dosage range of 250 to 400 milligrams a day for one week, there was a 50-percent increase in urinary excretion of C-2 estrogen. Increased urinary excretion is considered an indicator of increased production. It is feasible to increase production of C-2 estrogen with ingestion of 100 to 400 grams a day of raw cabbage or other cruciferous vegetables. Four cups of uncooked cabbage or broccoli can provide approximately 100 mg of I3C. It may be possible that a sizable increase in C-2 estrogen could take place with a smaller intake, according to the researchers at Strang Cornell Research Center, but this theory has not yet been tested. Indoles are made more available upon cooking.

Some substances will interfere with the process of breaking down estrogen into its C-2 form. The over-the-counter drug Tagamet (cimetidine), which blocks stomach acid secretions, decreases the amount of C-2 by 20 to 30 percent, thus increasing the amount of C-16 estrogen that is produced and slightly increasing breast-cancer risk.

There is a small percentage of women who don't produce the enzyme that will steer estrogen production toward the C-2 variety; no matter how many cruciferous vegetables they eat, they will make only C-16 estrogen.

KAEMPFEROL *(CAM-fer-awl)*. Kaempferol is a flavonoid phytochemical found in radishes and horseradish. Kaempferol is a powerful inhibitor of the cytochrome p450 system, which can activate cancer-causing substances.

LENTINAN *(LEN-tin-an)*. Lentinan is a phytochemical found in shiitake mushrooms that appears to have anticancer properties. In Japan, lentinan injected into patients, in combination with chemotherapeutic agents, has been successful in treating stomach, colorectal, and prostate cancer. Lentinan appears to stimulate increased production of biologically active serum factors associated with immunity and inflammation. Researchers report that it demonstrated remarkable lifespan-prolongation effects.

Lentinan is being studied also for its ability to fight the HIV virus. After four weeks of twice weekly oral administration of 1 milligram of lentinan, mice exhibited significantly higher levels of helper T-cells, which help other cells destroy infective organisms and lower levels of suppressor T-cells, which suppress the action of other immune cells, than did the mice in the control group. A human study of eleven adults who ingested 0.2 milligram of powdered lentinan daily revealed a higher percentage of active T-cells than those in the control group, who were not using the shiitake extract. It is reported that lentinan from shiitake mushrooms offers a potential treatment for HIV-positive individuals who are not too immunocompromised.

LIGNANS *(LIG-nenz)*. Lignan is a type of insoluble dietary fiber. Plant lignans are widely found in whole grains, legumes, and some vegetables, such as spinach, carrots, broccoli, and cauliflower. Flaxseeds also are noted for their lignan content. Flaxseed ground into meal has approximately thirty-seven times as much lignan as its nearest competitor, the lentil. Foods with modest lignan content are seaweed and oat bran. Lignans offer human beings the raw materials and the opportunity to create their own anticancer chemicals. These plant lignans first must be converted into mammalian lignans in the colon. When we ingest plant lignans, they are fermented in the colon and generate short-chain fatty acids that have the ability to act as a defense mechanism against cancer. The mammalian lignan bears a structural resemblance to estrogen and can bind to estrogen receptors, thus decreasing their uptake of circulating estrogen. Women who have breast cancer excrete low amounts of lignans in their urine, which scientists believe is indicative of diminished lignan circulation. The amount of lignan excretion can be increased eight to eighteen times by adding flaxseed powder to the diet of women with breast cancer, thus increasing the body content of lignan.

Depending upon a woman's estrogen status, lignans can either act as an estrogen-enhancing agent or as an anti-estrogen—guarding the cell against an estrogen overload. For premenopausal women with an abundance of estrogen, lignan will compete with circulating estrogen and decrease the amount of estrogen that the cell is exposed to. For menopausal or postmenopausal women who have low estrogen levels, the lignan will act like a source of estrogen, adding to the pool of circulating estrogenic substances, thereby working as an estrogen proxy.

LIGNINS (*LIG-ninz*). Lignins are structurally related to lignans, but they differ in their biological effects. Lignin is a type of insoluble dietary fiber that is found in the plant cell walls and can be resistant to breakdown by digestive enzymes.

LIMONENE (*LIGH-mo-neen*). Limonene, a monoterpene and phytochemical, is the simplest of the isoprenoids. It is found in citrus fruit oils and citrus fruit and in some herbs and spices, such as caraway, celery seed, cardamom, and fennel. Limonene has demonstrated the ability to impede the growth of skin, lung, breast, and stomach cancer in animal tests. When mice were treated with a known cancer-causing chemical, more than 80 percent of the chemically induced breast carcinomas completely regressed after treatment with limonene. Humans process limonene in a fashion similar to animals, so there is hope that it can be as effective for people. It appears to be both preventive and therapeutic.

Limonene works in a number of ways. It prevents the initiation of cancer. It also works during the promotion phase, and, more excitingly, it is effective on mammary tumor progression during full malignancy in animal studies. Researchers believe that limonene works as a blocking agent to prevent initiation of cancer by inducing enzyme systems that have the ability to deactivate known cancer-causing substances.

The therapeutic benefit of limonene may come from its ability to affect cell redifferentiation (the process of returning cells to their original specialized state). It has demonstrated this ability in cancers of the pancreas, prostate, and breast. When animals with mammary tumors were treated with limonene, the regressing tumor was remodeled from a carcinoma to a benign tumor.

Limonene is currently used in Japan to dissolve gallstones in doses of up to 20 grams per day with no known toxic effect.

Although limonene is found in citrus fruit oils and citrus fruits, the best sources of limonene are surprisingly not fruits but spices. Caraway is 3-percent limonene in dry weight, and celery seed is 2.5 percent. Oranges, cardamom, and fennel come in at slightly less than 1 percent (0.9 percent), and lime, spearmint, and nutmeg have 0.6 percent. Star anise and thyme have 0.5 percent.

LINALOL (*LIN-uh-lawl*). Linalol is found in grape leaves, lemon oil, thyme, coriander, winter savory, bergamot, and rosemary. It has anti-candida properties.

LINOLEIC (*lin-oh-LAY-ick*) **ACID.** Linoleic acid is an essential dietary polyunsaturated fatty acid found in the plant seeds, corn oil, and safflower oil. It is an omega-6 fatty acid. The human body uses linoleic acid to create anti-inflammatory prostaglandins but also can use it to make arachadonic acid, which in turn spawns prostaglandin 2 (PG2), which is found at the site of carcinomas.

LUTEIN (*LOO-teen*). Lutein, a member of the carotenoid family, is a dominant pigment in the macula of the eye. It is associated with a lower rate of age-related macular degeneration, which is the leading cause of blindness in the United States after age sixty-five. A 1994 Harvard University study showed that a daily intake of 6 milligrams of lutein was associated with a 43-percent lower incidence of age-related macular degeneration. Lutein is found predominantly in kale, spinach, parsley, and mustard greens.

LYCOPENE *(LIGH-co-peen)*. Lycopene is a carotenoid that displays powerful antioxidant activity. Lycopene exhibits twice the free-radical quenching ability of beta-carotene. It may exert its anticancer abilities by lending molecules to hungry free radicals that are created in the body in the course of normal metabolism. These free radicals will steal the molecule they need from the cell membrane if it is not in ready supply in the bloodstream. This loss from the cell membrane is thought to be the initial step in the development of heart disease or cancer. Lycopene is abundant in red and pink fruits and vegetables.

The richest known source of lycopene is canned tomato juice, but lycopene is more available to the body if it is cooked with some oil, so you will find an abundance of usable lycopene in spaghetti sauce. Other sources of lycopene are watermelon, guava, and pink grapefruit. Lycopene is scarce in other vegetables.

Lycopene may be the reason why men who ate ten or more servings a week of tomato products developed 45-percent fewer prostate cancers than men who ate fewer than two servings in a 1995 study of 47,000 health professionals. So it seems that eating ten or more servings weekly of tomatoes or other red or pink fruits may confer some protection against prostate cancer.

MONOUNSATURATED *(MAHN-o-un-SATCH-er-ate-ed)* **FATTY ACIDS.** Monounsaturated fatty acids are found naturally in abundance in fat-rich plant foods, such as olives and avocados. Canola oil, which is made from the rape plant, has been genetically engineered to have a high monounsaturated-fat content. These fatty acids are beneficial fats. Heart patients are often advised to substitute monounsaturated fats for polyunsaturated and saturated fats in their diets; some research shows them to improve the ratio of HDL to LDL cholesterol by raising HDL cholesterol (the "good" cholesterol). Increased intake of monounsaturated fats is sometimes indicated for people with diabetes because they can often help to stabilize insulin levels when a high-carbohydrate diet is ineffective. Although monounsaturated fats are thought to play a role in cancer prevention, their mode of action against cancer is unclear.

MYRICETIN *(mir-ISS-i-tin)*. Myricetin is a phytochemical found in ginger that has the ability to destroy the yeast candida.

NARINGENIN *(nar-IN-jin-in)*. Naringenin is a phytochemical found in large quantities in citrus fruits and in lesser amounts in the herbs oregano and tarragon. Dr. Duke's Phytochemical and Ethnobotanical database lists its biological activities as including working against HIV infection, blood platelet clumping, and tumor formation. It is also an inhibitor of the cytochrome p450 enzyme system; however, this biological activity had a negative effect in a group of grapefruit juice drinkers who also were taking the allergy medication Seldane. The naringenin in the grapefruit juice bound with the cytochrome p450 in the blood, thus decreasing the amount of cytochrome p450 available to degrade the Seldane. Seldane remained in the blood longer than expected, and as people continued to take the drug, Seldane levels became dangerously high. Seldane now comes with warning labels to avoid grapefruit and grapefruit juice due to its naringenin content.

PECTIN *(PEK-tin)*. Pectin is a soluble fiber found mostly in apples and citrus fruits. Soluble fibers have the ability to be fermented while in the colon. During the process of fermentation, they create butyrate, a fatty acid that has anticancer properties.

PERILLYL ALCOHOL *(PER-il-il AL-kuh-hawl)*. Perillyl alcohol is a potent monoterpene phytochemical found in cherries and in caraway seeds. It has demonstrated preventive and therapeutic properties against cancer. It is closely related to limonene, which is found in citrus fruits; however, perillyl alcohol is four to five times more powerful than limonene.

Perillyl alcohol appears to have the ability to induce apoptosis—programmed cell death in cancer cells. Perillyl alcohol found in cherries has demonstrated the ability to induce apoptosis and kill cancer cells during the promotion and progression phase of cancer in hamsters in which breast, colon, pancreatic, and liver cancers have been induced. When malignant tumors were transplanted into two groups of animals, those treated with perillyl alcohol showed a significant decrease in tumor growth, and 16 percent of the animals showed a complete regression of the tumors.

PHENYL ETHYL ISOTHIOCYNATE *(FEE-nil ETH-il IGH-so-THIGH-o-SIGH-nate)*. Phenyl ethyl isothiocynate (PEITC) is a phytochemical found in the entire family of cruciferous vegetables; however, watercress is the richest known source. PEITC demonstrates potent anticancer action, particularly in the lungs. In animal studies, when lung tumor growth was stimulated by a known carcinogen in cigarette smoke (4-methyl-nitrosamino)-1-(3-pyridyl)-1-butanone, more succinctly known as NNK, PEITC inhibited the growth of lung tumors by 50 percent. PEITC works by blocking the activation of NNK, the most potent cancer-causing substance found in cigarette smoke. NNK has to be activated by the phase I enzymes into its destructive form before it can enter the nucleus of the cell and interfere with the structure of DNA, eroding the code, which is the first step toward the initiation of cancer.

Animal and human studies show that the carcinogenic activity of NNK can be diminished by ingestion of PEITC. Dr. Stephen Hecht of the American Health Foundation in Valhalla, New York, a prominent researcher, states, "If you can't stop smoking, watercress helps to mitigate the effects of nicotine on lungs and will hopefully reduce incidence of lung cancer."

When Dr. Hecht and his colleagues fed 2 ounces of watercress to smokers three times a day, their urine samples were rich in the unactivated form of NNK. "It's most desirable for smokers to stop," Dr. Hecht stated, "but for addicted smokers, PEITC appears to be a highly promising compound for chemoprevention of lung cancer." Again, here is another phytochemical that works by blocking activation of cancer-causing substances.

PHTHALIDE *(THA-lide)*. Phthalide is a phytochemical found in the oil of the seed of the celery plant. Phthalide stimulates the activity of the glutathione-S-transferase enzyme system. When phthalide and sedanolide, another phytochemical found in celery, were tested on mice for their ability to inhibit a known cancer-causing substance, tumor incidence decreased from 68 percent in those not given anything to 30 percent in those treated with phthalide and 11 percent in those given sedanolide.

Phthalide also has demonstrated the ability to decrease the amount of catecholamines, hormones released in the blood in response to stress, when injected into animal subjects. Catecholamines cause blood vessels to constrict, which raises blood pressure. Researchers at the University of Chicago Medical Center have lowered blood pressure in lab animals by 12 to 14 percent by using this phytochemical found in celery.

PHYTOESTROGEN *(FIGH-to-ES-tro-jin)*. Phytoestrogens are estrogenlike compounds found in plants. Their intake leads to the production of estrogenlike substances, which can bind to estrogen receptors on cells and affect the way the genetic material expresses itself. Since estrogen exists only in the animal world, these compounds are not technically estrogens, but because of their chemical structure, they have the ability to act as weak estrogens.

Isoflavones, which are found largely in legumes and soy products, lead to the production of equol in some humans. Equol is a weak estrogen possessing about 0.2 percent of the biological activity of estradiol, one of the major estrogens found in humans. In the fruit world, both cherries and pomegranate seeds contain measurable amounts of phytoestrogen, but far less than the amounts detected in legumes. One researcher measured 1.7 milligrams of the phytoestrogen estrone in 3 ounces of pomegranate seeds. Lignans, which are found in wholegrain products and flaxseed oil, are also phytoestrogens.

Estrogen and phytoestrogen both bind to the cell on estrogen receptors, which are located on the outside of the estrogen-sensitive cell. Phytoestrogens can work in two ways, depending upon the estrogen status of the woman. In the premenopausal woman, they can compete with the body's own estrogen for attachment to the estrogen receptors, thus diminishing the amount of genuine estrogen that enters the cell. In the postmenopausal woman, they can serve as a source of estrogen and bind to estrogen receptors, thus enhancing the effects of estrogen. Phytoestrogens may act as antagonists to hormone-dependent cancers (breast, cervical, and endometrial), which are fueled by human estrogen, but their use is controversial for postmenopausal women because of their weak estrogenic abilities. They are often thought of as good estrogens because they are less potent than a woman's own estrogen.

QUERCETIN *(KERS-a-tin)*. Quercetin is a member of the bioflavonoid family, and it is found in red grapes, berries, tomatoes, potatoes, pea pods, and onions with colored skins. In laboratory tests, scientists isolated breast cancer cells from human tissue, and quercetin was highly effective in inhibiting the growth of these cancers. In a study of breast cancer cells that were not estrogen dependent, quercetin inhibited tumor growth by 50 percent after three days of exposure. It also has shown effectiveness in inhibiting leukemia cells, squamous cell carcinoma that originated in the head and neck, gastric and colon cancer, and both estrogen-dependent and estrogen-independent cancers. It is thought that the growth-inhibitory effects of quercetin may be a consequence of its ability to interfere with enzyme systems that regulate cell proliferation. Quercetin also has the ability to inhibit LDL cholesterol oxidation, which is the first step in the process of the development of cardiovascular disease.

RESVERATROL *(res-VER-a-trol)*. Resveratrol is a phytochemical found in grapes that has proven to be effective against cancer in cell and animal studies. It inhibits cancer initiation, promotion, and progression: the three major stages of cancer development.

SAPONINS *(SAY-pun-inz)*. Saponins are phytochemicals found in legumes, most notably soybeans. They have the ability to combine oil and water, which helps them bind to cholesterol and increase its excretion from the body. They also appear to have anticancer properties, as they interfere with the process by which DNA reproduces. This may prevent cancer cells from multiplying.

SEDANOLIDE *(se-DAN-o-LIDE)*. Sedanolide is a phytochemical found in celery that stimulates the activity of the glutathione-S-transferase enzyme system. Along with phthalide, sedanolide is found in the oil of the seed of the celery plant and is responsible for its characteristic odor.

SELENIUM *(se-LEEN-ee-um)*. Selenium is a mineral that can be found in plant foods. The selenium content of the soil the food is grown in dictates the amount of selenium that will be found in the food. Selenium-rich soil will grow selenium-rich food. Whole grains can be a good source of selenium, depending upon the selenium content of the soil in which they were grown. Selenium is an essential cofactor for the enzyme glutathione peroxidase, which disarms dangerous peroxide molecules. The enzyme acts as an antioxidant within the matrix of the cell preventing free-radical damage. Selenium deficiency can lead to an enlarged heart and ultimately heart failure.

Selenium is present in very low doses in common foods. Diets that are high in selenium have been shown to suppress the induction of cancer in a variety of animal studies. It is believed that selenium works to prevent the initiation and possibly the progression of cancer. Cancer patients often have low levels of selenium in their blood. High doses of selenium are toxic. The recommended intake for selenium for men and women is 70 and 55 micrograms, respectively.

SHOGAOL *(sho-JAHL)*. Shogaol is a phytochemical found in the ginger plant that acts as an antitussive to prevent coughing. It also has anti-inflammatory properties.

SILYMARIN *(SIL-lee-MAR-en)*. Silymarin is classified as a flavonoid phytochemical. It is found in artichokes, as well as in the milk thistle plant. It offers anticancer protection through its ability to act as an antioxidant. In a study done at Case Western Reserve University in Cleveland in 1994, dermatologists applied silymarin at various dose levels to the skin of mice. They then applied known tumor-promoting chemicals. They measured the activity of a biochemical marker, which indicates tumor promotion. They found that topical application of 2 milligrams of silymarin resulted in the complete inhibition of tumor activity.

Silymarin also is known for its effectiveness in the treatment of alcohol-induced liver disorders. Real improvement of liver function has been attributed to treatment with 420 milligrams a day of silymarin. Double-blind controlled studies measured the liver function of people with mildly acute liver disorders who admitted drinking on a

59

daily basis. Those treated with silymarin showed improvement in their liver function tests more rapidly than those receiving the placebo.

In other studies, animals pretreated with silymarin who were then exposed to a wide range of known liver toxins had less liver damage than those animals who were not treated with silymarin. Many scientists believe that silymarin offers potential as a chemoprotective agent against a wide range of toxins.

STEVIOSIDE *(STEE-vee-oh-SIDE)*. Stevioside is a sweet crystalline form of glucose extracted from the leaf of the *Stevia rebaudiana,* a small shrub found in Paraguay. It is approximately 300 times sweeter than table sugar. It has been used as a sweetener in Paraguay for over 100 years and is currently used as a sweetening agent in Japan, China, Korea, Taiwan, Israel, Uruguay, and Paraguay. The best-tasting whole leaf stevia is said to be harvested from its native habitat, and cultivating it away from its indigenous soil results in an off-taste that is biting and metallic, making the taste of stevia variable depending upon its origin.

Stevia has not been approved for use by the United States Food and Drug Administration as a sweetener, but it is imported into the United States as a dietary supplement. Standards for dietary supplements, which are not as stringent as the standards for food additives, are controlled by the Dietary Supplement Health and Education Act, regulated under the Food, Drug and Cosmetic Act. Proponents of stevia as a dietary supplement claim that it can lower blood pressure, strengthen the heart and vascular system, boost immunity, improve digestion, reduce weight, clear up skin problems, act as a contraceptive, and enhance youthfulness. Scanty evidence is available on the validity of these claims.

STIGMASTEROL *(STIG-muh-STER-awl)*. Stigmasterol is a phytosterol that is found in beans and bean and seed oils. It may be useful in treating benign hyperplasia of the prostate gland.

SULFORAPHANE *(Sul-FOR-uh-FANE)*. Sulforaphane is found in cruciferous vegetables and in vegetable sprouts. It has been shown to reduce breast tumor formation in rats that were treated with a known carcinogen. The animals that were fed more sulphoraphane developed fewer tumors. This is what scientists refer to as a dose-related response. Sulforaphane inhibits the activation of carcinogens. Scientists are very excited about sulforaphane and its potential as a chemoprotective agent.

THYMOL *(THIGH-mawl).* Thymol is a phytochemical found in lemons, thyme, bergamot, and rosemary. It is listed in Dr. Duke's phytochemical database as having anti-Alzheimer's properties. It also has anti-dental-plaque, anticavity, and other dental health properties.

TOCOTRIENOLS *(TO-ko-TREE-in-awls).* Tocotrienols are phytochemicals that have potent isoprenoid activity. The tocotrienols are found in a variety of fruits, vegetables, and whole grains. Notable amounts have been detected in barley, oats, and alfalfa. They help to lengthen the dormant stage of tumor cells and decrease the proliferation of tumors. They also are helpful in controlling serum cholesterol.

TUMERIN *(TOO-mer-in).* Tumerin is a phytochemical compound found in turmeric. It is a strong antioxidant and protects DNA from oxidative injury.

ZEAXANTHIN *(ZEE-uh-ZAN-thin).* Zeaxanthin is a phytochemical isolated from deep green vegetables like kale, collard greens, spinach, Swiss chard, mustard greens, and okra, romaine lettuce, and red pepper. Zeaxanthin forms the yellow pigment in the eye, and its intake is thought to prevent macular degeneration.

ZINGERONE *(ZIN-jer-one).* Zingerone is a phytochemical isolated from the ginger plant that has antioxidant and anti-inflammatory properties.

So, as you can see, phytochemicals are numerous and varied in their functions—and this is just the tip of the iceberg. There are hundreds more phytochemicals still being studied and yet to be discovered. While not yet considered by scientists to be necessary for the sustenance of human life, it is clear that they play a vital role in the maintenance of good health.

4

The Most Powerful Foods

This chapter will be your guide to the most phytochemically dense foods. From this roster of foods, you will learn where to find and how to maximize all of the well-known phytochemicals. After reading the previous chapters, you know what phytochemicals are and what they do. This chapter will now direct you to the foods richest in these phytochemicals. All plant foods contain phytochemicals, but some appear to contain more than others.

This information was gathered to provide you with the facts you need to focus your food selection on supporting and maintaining your well-being. Included in this section is information about selecting, preparing, and storing foods in order to maximize phytochemical intake.

The study of phytochemicals as they pertain to health is a work in progress, so definitive information about amounts of foods or phytochemicals needed to obtain perceived benefits is not always available. Where that information is available, every effort was made to include it. Hopefully at some time in the future, the phytochemical content of foods will be included among nutrition information prepared and distributed by the United States Department of Agriculture so that we can make better-informed choices about our food selections.

THE PHYTOCHEMICAL MAKEUP OF FOODS

Certain phytochemicals are widely distributed in foods, and it is safe to assume that they will be found in almost all fruits and vegetables to some extent; thus they are not mentioned individually in the discussions of each fruit and vegetable. One of the most commonly found phytochemicals is chlorogenic acid, which is found in the highest amounts in freshly harvested fruits and vegetables. The phenolic compounds caffeic and ferulic acids are also widely distributed in foods, and you can ensure an adequate intake by eating a wide variety of fresh fruits and vegetables. On the other hand, although certain phytochemicals are typically found in certain foods, there is no guarantee that they will be present. Plant genetics is believed to play a major role in the phytochemical content of food. Different varieties of the same food have been found to have vastly different phytochemical contents.

Growing conditions also may play a role in the phytochemical makeup of foods. There is a story told about broccoli that was grown on the upward and downward slopes of a hill in Israel. One side of the hill yielded vegetables rich in indoles; the broccoli from the opposing side was void of the same phytochemicals.

SELECTING AND PREPARING YOUR PHYTOCHEMICAL-RICH PRODUCE

When shopping for fruits and vegetables, remember that locally grown produce is more likely to be fresh than produce that has traveled a long distance to reach you, so you may maximize your chlorogenic acid intake by eating locally grown produce in season.

If at all practical, leave the edible skins on fruits and vegetables when eating them. Much of the phytochemical content of produce is often found in the skin. For example, the flavonoid phytochemical quercetin is located in the highest amounts in the outer layers of fruits and vegetables. Wash the fruit and vegetables thoroughly, a vegetable brush works well, and cut away any bruised or damaged areas. The phytochemical content of canned fruits and vegetables, which are often peeled, may be diminished. You will be maximizing the available phytochemicals by eating clean edible plant skins.

Phytochemicals can be very volatile. Cooking and puréeing have been shown to make certain phytochemicals more available for absorption by the body. Simple processing like the crushing of garlic alters this food's phytochemical content, and vigorous chewing of broccoli and the other cruciferous vegetables greatly improves the likelihood that indoles will form. Where applicable, I will tell you which fruits' and vegetables' phytochemical content is increased with processing.

Organic produce, which is grown without the use of harmful pesticides or other chemicals, is the best source of phytochemicals, particularly when diet is being used as a treatment for a disease such as cancer. When pesticides are ingested, the body will be called upon to work harder to process and detoxify them. Researchers frequently use pesticides to create cancer in lab animals to measure the effectiveness of their hypothetical cure. If you are fighting cancer, it makes sense to avoid substances that cause cancer. A healthy person may have the ability to process and excrete pesticides with minimal damage, but a person who is trying to direct his or her biological energy toward healing would be wise to minimize added biological stress.

Finally, before you eat, take time to appreciate and enjoy the bounty of food that nature has set before you.

ALMONDS. *See* Nuts and Seeds.

APPLES

Apples are good sources of the plant fiber pectin. Pectin is useful for controlling high cholesterol. Apples are also sources of quercetin and ascorbic acid. A wide variety of fresh apples are available year-round. Apples also are available dried, canned, and jarred as applesauce; however, since the peels have been removed, the phytochemical content of canned apples and applesauce will be less than that of fresh apples. Dried apples are good choices, as long as the peel has not been removed. When choosing fresh fruit, select tight-skinned, unblemished fruits. Keep apples in the refrigerator for storage to retain the crispness of the fruit. Remove them shortly before eating to bring the fruit to room temperature in order to maximize its taste.

APRICOTS

Apricots are good sources of beta-carotene and fiber. The people of the Hunza—a remote little kingdom high in the Himalayas—have attracted scientific and media attention because of their superb health and longevity. A staple of their diet is apricots. Fresh apricots are available from June through August from the northeastern United States, but they are fragile. They are ready to eat if the flesh yields to the slight pressure of a squeeze. Dried and canned apricots are available year-round.

ARTICHOKES

Artichokes are a source of silymarin—the average artichoke contains about 6 milligrams. Silymarin has antioxidant and anticancer properties and is known for its effectiveness in the treatment of alcohol-induced liver disease. Artichokes are also a fair source of folic acid and a good source of the anticancer polyphenols that are found abundantly in green tea. Artichokes are available fresh, or artichoke hearts can be bought frozen, canned, and jarred. Drain canned and jarred artichoke hearts before using. They make a good addition to salads, and the marinated hearts serve up quickly, sliced and topped with a pimento on crackers as a premeal snack.

ARUGULA

Arugula is a member of the family of cruciferous vegetables and contains the phytochemicals sulforaphane, indole-3-carbinol, dithiolthione, isothiocynate, and all the other phytochemicals that are specific to the family of cruciferous vegetables. When it's sold in seed packages, arugula is sometimes called roquette or rocket. It is a spicy leafy green vegetable that grows easily in the garden or a terrace pot. It's sold fresh in bunches in the supermarket or green market, and it's often included in prepared salad mixtures that are sold by the pound fresh in the produce section. Adding arugula to salad greens is a good way of including cruciferous vegetables in your diet if you have not yet developed a taste for cooked cabbage or broccoli, or if you just want to increase your intake of cruciferous vegetables.

Asparagus

Asparagus contains asparagus crude saponins, which inhibited the growth of human leukemia cells in a study done at Rutgers University. It also acts as a diuretic. Asparagus is also a source of folic acid, carotenoids, and vitamin E. Fresh asparagus is most abundant in the spring, but it is available canned and frozen throughout the year. Select fresh asparagus for their uniform thickness so they cook consistently. Wash and snap off the woody ends before cooking.

Avocados

Avocados are fruit that are rich sources of the phytochemical mono-unsaturated fatty acid. They also contain vitamin E, folic acid, and fiber, along with other essential nutrients. They are available year-round. The two states that provide us with avocados are Florida and California. From California, we get Haas avocados, which are small and pear-shaped with a thick pebble skin that turns black when ripe. One ounce of Haas avocado has 5 grams of fat, 73 percent of which is from monounsaturated fatty acids. From Florida, we get larger smooth-skinned avocados that are a brighter green and rounder in shape. The Florida avocados, whose skins do not blacken as they grow ripe, have less oil than the California variety. One ounce of Florida avocado contains 2.5 grams of fat, and 61 percent of the fat content is from monounsaturated fatty acids. Both varieties are ready for eating when they yield to slight pressure.

Bananas

Bananas come to us from tropical climates and are America's most favorite fruit. Due to their smooth texture, they can be enjoyed by the very young and by people who have problems chewing. They are fair sources of beta-carotene and are among the few fruits that contain the phytochemical fructooligosaccharide, which is a sweet-tasting nutritional fiber that appears to be useful in maintaining a healthy balance of bacteria in the colon. Bananas are among the few fruits that ripen as well or better off the plant than on it. They are available year-round.

BARLEY

Barley is an ancient grain that was a favorite in Victorian times. It has fallen somewhat out of fashion in American cuisine, but it is used frequently as a soup ingredient. Barley cereal is one of the first grains that we feed babies because it is easy to digest due to its lack of gluten. In addition to being a good source of fiber, it's also a fairly good source of carotenoids and vitamin E. The soluble fiber in barley makes it good for controlling cholesterol, and it is thought to have a measure of anticancer activity as well. Barley can be cooked with water like rice to make a side dish or combined with beans for a main dish.

BEANS

There are dozens of varieties of beans, including adzuki beans, black beans, chick peas, fava beans, Great Northern beans, lentils, lima beans, and pinto beans, just to name a few. In addition to being a significant source of the amino acids that make up protein, they contain fiber, vitamins, and minerals. Beans also are stocked with protease inhibitors, phytosterols, saponins, and isoflavones, all potent phytochemicals that inhibit a multitude of diseases. Yellow split peas and lima beans are excellent sources of genistein, and pinto beans are a great source of daidzein. A one-half-cup serving of beans daily will deliver a significant amount of all these beneficial phytochemicals.

Beans are available dried or canned. Dried beans are less expensive than canned beans, but they require cooking before they can be eaten. Most beans need to be soaked before they are cooked with the exception of split peas, lentils, and lima beans.

BERRIES

Among the many varieties of berries, blackberries, blueberries, cranberries, raspberries, and strawberries are good sources of the anticancer phytochemicals anthocyanin, ellagic acid, and carotenoids. Berries are also rich in quercetin, which is thought to protect against cardiovascular disease as well as cancer, and they are a good source of the phytonutrient ascorbic acid. Most berries are also very good sources of fiber. Blueberries are particularly rich in antioxidant activity. One cup of blueberries alone supplies a whopping 3,200 ORAC units (see page 12). Strawberries are not quite as potent as blueberries but also offer significant protection against free radicals in test-tube studies. Fresh berries are most abundant in late spring through late summer, but frozen and canned berries are available all year long. Frozen berries are available unsweetened but are more often sold commercially heavily sugared. Try to avoid these.

BLACKBERRIES. *See* Berries.

BLUEBERRIES. *See* Berries.

BRAZIL NUTS. *See* Nuts and Seeds.

BROCCOLI

Broccoli is a member of the family of cruciferous vegetables, which provide a wealth of phytochemicals, including sulforaphane, indole-3-carbinol, dithiolethione, and isothiocynate. In addition to the assortment of phytochemicals that are common to all cruciferous vegetables, broccoli is also a source of beta-carotene, folic acid, quercetin, ascorbic acid, protease inhibitors, lutein, and calcium. The calcium that is present in broccoli is better absorbed by the body than the calcium from milk—32 percent of the calcium present in milk is absorbed by the body compared with 53 percent of the calcium from broccoli. The indole-3-carbinol and beta-carotene from broccoli are made more available for absorption after cooking. Broccoli is available year-round, fresh and frozen, and it can be eaten raw or cooked. Select broccoli for its dark green color and velvety firmly packed head. Yellow florets are a sign of age and toughness in broccoli and should be avoided. In addition to being sold in heads, broccoli is also available in florets at the salad bar. Broccoli florets are perfect when you need only a small amount of broccoli—that is, when cooking for one, or when it is used in a medley of vegetables in a stir-fry.

BROCCOLI SPROUTS

Broccoli sprouts are immature broccoli plants that are produced by sprouting broccoli seeds. In general, sprouts resemble the food of their origin in nutritive value but contain increased amounts of vitamins A and C, less carbohydrate, and more protein than the mature product. Broccoli sprouts have been reported to contain thirty to fifty times more sulforaphane than mature broccoli, according to researchers at Johns Hopkins Medical Center. Broccoli sprouts are generally available in natural foods stores, though they have been showing up lately in some supermarkets as well, or they can be made in your own kitchen. For step-by-step sprouting information, try reading *American Wholefoods Cuisine* by David and Nikki Goldbeck. If you choose to sprout your own seeds, it is essential that you select untreated vegetable seeds. Many packaged garden seeds are treated with fungicides.

BRUSSELS SPROUTS

Brussels sprouts look like tiny individual heads of cabbage. They are available fresh and frozen year-round. They are members of the cruciferous vegetable family, and they contribute sulforaphane, indole-3-carbinol, dithiolethione, and isothiocynates to the diet. In addition, Brussels sprouts are good sources of the anticancer protease inhibitors, beta-carotene, and vitamin E.

CABBAGE

Cabbage is a member of the family of cruciferous vegetables, which is packed with some of the most potent disease-fighting phytochemicals. The phytochemicals available from cabbage include dithiolethione, isothiocynate, indole-3-carbinol, and sulforaphane. In addition, cabbage is a source of ascorbic acid, folic acid, and the carotenoids. It is available fresh in the produce section of the supermarket in many varieties. Red cabbage is also a source of the phytochemical anthocyanin. Sauerkraut is cabbage that has been preserved in brine. Since the cancer-fighting indoles in cruciferous vegetables are more available after being heated, cooked cabbage might be a better source of indole-3-carbinol than uncooked cabbage dishes like cole slaw. Researchers were able to increase the production of anti-breast-cancer estrogen metabolites in women by feeding them four cups of uncooked cabbage. It's likely that less-cooked cabbage would achieve the same result, since cooking makes the indoles more available. The high fiber content of cabbage makes it a good addition to the diet to alleviate constipation. Researchers estimate that approximately one cup of cooked caggage can deliver about 100 milligrams of indole-3-carbinol.

CANTALOUPE

Cantaloupe is a significant source of the antioxidant phytochemical beta-carotene, as are most orange-colored flesh fruits, excluding oranges. In fact, one cup of cantaloupe delivers just under half of one's daily requirement of beta-carotene. Cantaloupes are ripe when the stem end is soft and when the green webbing of its skin has faded to beige or yellow. The tastiest cantaloupes also have a fragrance. Avoid melons that have scars or mold on them. Store them at home at room temperature until ripe. When the melon is ripened, cut it up and store in the refrigerator in a covered bowl or plastic container. The peak time for cantaloupe availability is May through the early fall. Melon balls also can be purchased frozen. Serve these partially thawed. If allowed to thaw completely, they become mushy.

CARAWAY SEEDS

The herb caraway is a member of the carrot family. The seeds are among the richest known sources of the cancer-fighting phytochemical limonene. Caraway is 3-percent limonene by dry weight. A teaspoon of caraway seeds mixed in with a brick of low-fat cream cheese will boost the phytochemical content of your basic bagel-and-cream-cheese breakfast. Caraway seeds are often found on rye bread.

CARROTS

Carrots and other vegetables with a deep orange color contain large quantities of beta-carotene. Two factors that can impact the absorption of beta-carotene from carrots and other beta-carotene-rich foods are particle size and heat. The amount of beta-carotene absorbed from raw carrots can be as little as 1 to 2 percent. Application of heat to the carrots seems to increase the biological availability of beta-carotene and hence increases the amount absorbed by the body. About one cooked carrot delivers two times the RDA for beta-carotene.

The particle size of uncooked food is also important; puréed or finely chopped vegetables result in considerably higher beta-carotene absorption compared with whole or sliced raw vegetables. Carrots are available fresh, canned, and frozen year-round.

CASHEWS. *See* Nuts and Seeds.

CAULIFLOWER

Cauliflower is a member of the cruciferous family of vegetables. It is a good source of ascorbic acid, indoles, and isothiocynates. Select produce with a firm, compact head with creamy white flowerets and bright green leaves.

CELERY

Phthalide and sedanolide are phytochemicals found in celery and are responsible for the distinctive smell of celery and its anticancer capabilities. Phthalide also is recognized for its ability to lower blood pressure. Celery and celery oil have been used in East Asian folk medicine for centuries to treat high blood pressure, which is surprising since the sodium content of celery is relatively high for a vegetable. Researchers were able to lower blood pressure in animals by 12 to 14 percent by feeding them a small quantity of phthalide. An equivalent amount of phthalide for a person can be obtained from about four stalks of celery. The university-based researcher, Qang T. Lee, undertook this study after his father demonstrated that he could lower his blood pressure by this simple technique. Celery is also a source of ascorbic acid, folic acid, and vitamin E. Celery is available fresh all year in the produce section of the supermarket. Avoid bunches that have cracked and bruised stalks. Stalks with air holes in the central portion, sometimes caused by frost, are undesirable.

CHERRIES

Cherries are among the few known food sources of the potent anticancer phytochemical perillyl alcohol. Perillyl alcohol is noted for its selective effect to induce cell death in tumor cells without affecting normal benign cells. This is an extremely desirable trait to come upon in a food because this is exactly the effect the ideal chemotherapy drug would induce. Though, according to Dr. Pamela Crowell, a researcher in the forefront of perillyl alcohol research, one cannot eat enough cherries to achieve high enough doses of perillyl alcohol to mimic the effects of chemotherapy drugs, one can receive anticancer benefits from eating average amounts of cherries. Cherries are also rich in anthocyanins and quercetin and are good sources of the phytonutrients ascorbic acid and fiber. Cherries are available fresh most abundantly in the summer but also are sold in cans and jars on supermarket shelves all year long.

CHICK PEAS. *See* Beans.

CITRUS FRUITS

The oil of citrus fruits, which includes grapefruits, oranges, lemons, limes, and tangerines, is a good source of the monoterpene phytochemical limonene. It is also an excellent source of the plant form of vitamin C—ascorbic acid—and the fiber pectin. Folic acid also is found in small quantities in orange juice. Carotenoids, coumaric acid, and phenol phytochemicals also can be obtained from citrus fruit.

Grapefruit and oranges contain naringenin, a phytochemical that binds to the enzyme cytochrome p450 in the cell, making the cytochrome p450 less available for other tasks. Pink grapefruit also contains the phytochemical lycopene, a powerful antioxidant.

When selecting citrus fruits, remember that thin-skinned fruits that feel heavy for their size will have more juice than thick-skinned fruits. The white, or albedo, of the citrus fruit contains glucarates and bioflavonoids. Bioflavonoids are biologically active flavonoids that work synergistically with vitamin C and provide the raw materials needed by

Limonene-ade

To maximize the amount of phytochemicals available from organic citrus fruit: Dice the rinds of two or three pieces of organic citrus fruit, cover with two to three cups of water, and boil. Strain. Add maple syrup or honey to taste to the hot mixture. Refrigerate. Serve over ice.

the body to create the connective tissue necessary for healing. When peeling or juicing citrus fruit, try to leave some of the albedo on the fruit to maximize its phytochemical content.

COLLARD GREENS

Collard greens are members of the family of cruciferous vegetables, which can provide the phytochemicals sulforaphane, indole-3-carbinol, dithiolethione, isothiocynate, lutein, and zeaxanthin. In addition, they are excellent sources of the phytonutrients beta-carotene and calcium. In one cup of collard greens there are 5 grams of fiber, 225 milligrams of calcium, and more than half of a daily supply of vitamin C and beta-carotene. They are available fresh year-round with the peak season being December to March. They are also sold frozen. Add well-washed, roughly chopped collards, whose tough mid-rib has been removed, to a saucepan with an inch of boiling water. Bring to a rapid boil. Cover and simmer until tender. Drain and season, reserving the liquid, often called the "pot licker." Traditionally in the South, the pot licker is served with corn bread.

CORN

Corn contains protease inhibitors, which possess anticancer capabilities. Yellow corn, but not white corn, contains a meager amount of carotenoid activity. All corn is a good source of fiber. Corn is available fresh, frozen, and canned, as well as dry as popcorn.

CRANBERRIES. *See* Berries.

CUCUMBERS

Cucumbers contain protease inhibitors, which have anticancer properties. Cucumbers are available fresh in a number of varieties, all equally phytochemically rich. They also are sold as pickles bottled in brine.

CUMIN

Cumin is a spice that reportedly has anticancer activities. Cumin is found in at least two varieties: black cumin and yellow-brown cumin. Both are used in Indian cooking, but the yellow-brown variety seems to predominate around the world. The ethnobotanist James Duke reports that cumin contains carveol and limonene among its assortment of anticancer phytochemicals.

According to a retrospective study conducted at the Western Gailee Regional Hospital in Israel of 964 patients of the urology department: Those patients that had consumed the most water, the most olive oil, and the most cumin were the least likely to develop prostate cancer.

FENNEL

Fennel is a member of the carrot family. This vegetable also is used as an herb. It is a good source of the anticancer monoterpene limonene. It is sold fresh in the produce section of the grocery store, and the seeds are sold dried for brewing tea. Fresh fennel can be sliced into a salad. It's used most notably in Italian cookery in the making of soups.

Fennel seeds can be used as a carminative (inducer of gas expulsion) and as a diuretic. They are highly regarded by the noted herbalist Culpeper for their ability to "expel wind and provoke urine." Fennel leaves and seeds also are thought to increase the flow and the quality of mother's milk when boiled with barley water.

FIGS

Fig trees originated in the Mediterranean region. The Hebrew Torah mentions figs for their ability to heal. Fresh figs are available in the spring and summer months. Dried figs are a significant source of cal-

It's Like Comparing Apples and Dried Apples

Ounce for ounce, dried fruit sometimes appears more phytochemically dense than the same variety of fresh fruit. That's because the water content of fresh fruit is higher, which adds more weight. So when they're examined side by side ounce for ounce for phytonutrients (except ascorbic acid) and phytochemicals, the dried fruit will appear to deliver more. Bear in mind that ounce for ounce, the same weight of dried fruit also will have a higher sugar content and more calories than the fresh fruit.

cium. Ten dried figs have 269 milligrams of calcium, slightly shy of the amount of calcium delivered by an 8-ounce serving of dairy food. Figs are also a significant source of fiber.

FLAXSEEDS

Flaxseeds are tiny brown egg-shaped seeds that are silken to the touch and notable for two reasons; one is their lignan content. Lignans are phytochemicals that have the ability to mimic estrogen. Sometimes they are called phytoestrogens. The other notable feature of flaxseeds is their high content of the omega-3 fatty acids, which are also found in fish. Flaxseeds also contain flavonoids, coumaric acid, and phenolic phytochemicals.

The benefits of flaxseed can be made available upon grinding the flaxseed into meal or flour. The flax flour can then be used in recipes as a substitute for 10 percent of the total wheat flour content without negatively altering the taste of the recipe. The flax flour will provide a nutty flavor to the product. The ground flaxseed also can be sprinkled in yogurt or on breakfast cereal. A small electric coffee bean grinder works well for grinding the flaxseeds into meal. Flaxseeds are sold in natural food stores.

In research done on healthy volunteers in Canada, 50 grams (almost 2 ounces) of flax flour taken as a supplement or incorporated into baked products lowered total cholesterol in the participants by 9 percent and LDL cholesterol (the so-called "bad" cholesterol) by 18 percent without affecting HDL cholesterol (the so-called "good" cholesterol). When 50 grams of flax flour was substituted for 50 grams of an alternate carbohydrate, the post-meal blood-glucose response in healthy volunteers was decreased by 27 percent, suggesting that flaxseed might be useful when substituted for other carbohydrates in a diet designed to control diabetes.

Flaxseed oil is one of the richest known plant sources of omega-3 fatty acids, but it is almost devoid of lignans. You can, however, purchase a flaxseed oil with added lignans. It takes three tablespoons of flax meal to equal the concentration of omega-3 fatty acids in one teaspoon of flaxseed oil. Heat, light, and oxygen are enemies of flaxseed oil, which makes flaxseed oil inappropriate for use at the high temperatures needed for frying and grilling. The seeds, as well as the oil, should be refrigerated between uses. Milled (ground) flaxseed has been stored at room temperature for up to four months (128 days) without any noticeable changes in flavor. In one study, after 128 days, minor amounts of the oxidation by-product hexanol were present in the flaxseed, which indicated that the oils had been somewhat deteriorated by oxidation.

GARLIC

Garlic is a member of the allium family of vegetables to which onions also belong. Garlic contains the phytochemicals ajoene and allicin. Ajoene is responsible for garlic's ability to make blood platelets less sticky. Allicin is a sulfide phytochemical that is principally responsible for garlic's ability to lower cholesterol, lower blood pressure, and possibly reduce the risk of stomach cancer. Noted phytochemical researcher Dr. Mike Wargovich advises that "constant exposure to allium vegetables in the diet protects against cancer." Garlic also contains monoterpene and phenolic phytochemicals. About two cloves of raw or slightly cooked garlic will probably confer benefits.

You'll notice that an uncut clove of garlic sitting on the kitchen counter has no odor. Allicin, which is responsible for many of garlic's healthful qualities, also is responsible for its odor. To release the power of allicin, garlic needs to be cut or bruised. The more cuts in the garlic, the more allicin is released. When using fresh garlic, crushed garlic will be most potent; minced and sliced come in second and third. Garlic can be eaten raw but may be irritating to sensitive stomachs. When cooking with garlic, to maximize the phytochemical content, add the garlic shortly before the dish is finished cooking. Garlic is available fresh, bottled, or powdered. The elephant variety of garlic is milder in flavor, perhaps due to its lack of ajoene. Researchers have measured as much allicin in one-third of a teaspoon of garlic powder as appears in most garlic-supplement pills.

GINGER

Ginger is a culinary herb whose phytochemicals are useful for a wide variety of disorders. Ginger contains the phytochemicals gingerol, shogaol, and zingerone, all of which are antioxidants. Gingerol is listed in the United States Department of Agriculture's phytochemical database as an antiemetic, which means that it acts to prevent nausea and vomiting. It's no wonder that ginger ale has long been a favorite home remedy for a queasy stomach. Ginger is used in Europe for morning sickness and for the nausea associated with motion sickness. It also is useful as a decongestive remedy. The phytochemicals gingerol and shogaol act as antitussives, which means they are useful for the congestion associated with colds and flu.

Ginger can be used dried or grated fresh; there's no need to remove the papery peel. It's also sold in crystalline form as a candy. Ginger is best taken with food, as it can cause heartburn if taken on an empty stomach.

The zingerone and the shogaol found in ginger have anti-inflammatory properties. Ginger makes a useful alternative to nonsteroidal anti-inflammatory drugs (NSAIDs), which are responsible for 20,000 deaths a year and 20 percent of the ulcers that are diagnosed. Noted doctor of alternative medicine Dr. Andrew Weil recommends one capsule of dried ginger twice a day for the treatment of musculoskeletal conditions like arthritis and fibromyalgia.

The phytochemicals in ginger also appear to confer protection from cancer by increasing glutathione-S-transferase production. Studies show that ginger oil suppresses changes in a cell's DNA that can be caused by the mold aflatoxin B_1. The ginger oil appears to inhibit the enzymes that activate aflatoxin B_1 and cause carcinogens to form. This would make ginger most effective as an inhibitor of cancer.

GRAPES

Grapes contain the phytochemicals resveratrol and ellagic acid, and quercetin, as well as some phytosterols. Concord grapes are workhorses at disarming free-radical molecules in test tubes, according to the scientists at the United States Department of Agriculture Human Nutrition Center on Aging, where they are testing various foods for their Oxygen Radical Absorbance Capacity (ORAC—see page 12). There are about 800 ORAC units in 3.5 ounces of grapes. Raisins, which are dried grapes, provide more than 2,800 ORAC units in a similar serving. Scientists suggest that 3,000 to 5,000 ORAC units are needed daily to offer a significant protective effect against disease.

Dr. John Folts of the University of Wisconsin Medical School has found that drinking 10 ounces a day of purple grape juice makes blood platelets less sticky and less likely to form the blood clots that can lead to heart attacks. Grape juice is more effective than aspirin for its ability to inhibit blood from forming clots. Aspirin slows the activity of platelets by 45 percent, whereas grape juice slows them by 75 percent.

It has been known for almost a decade that the French, who eat diets high in saturated fat but drink red wine daily, have a lower mortality rate from cardiovascular disease than Americans. It is probable that they are afforded protection by the flavonoid content of the wine, making their blood platelets less sticky. Now we know that we may be able to get the same effect without the addition of alcohol to our diets by drinking purple grape juice.

GREEN TEA

Green tea is widely consumed in Asia in quantities that equal the amount of coffee consumed in America. It has a mild, yet distinctive, flavor compared with other teas and coffee. The difference between green tea and the black tea that Americans are more familiar with is the amount of fermentation that they have undergone. Black tea is made from green tea leaves that have been fermented by allowing them to sit and generate their own internal heat. This heat changes the look, the taste, and the chemical structure of the tea.

Green tea is a source of the phenolic phytochemical epigallocatechin-3-gallate (EGCG), which has the ability to interfere with the process of cancer at all stages of its development. EGCG is also a significant cholesterol-lowering agent. Green tea also contains flavonoids, glucarates, and coumarins. The antioxidants in green tea are 100 times more effective than vitamin C and 25 times better than vitamin E at protecting cells from damage that can potentially cause cancer, heart disease, and other illnesses.

Drinking four cups of green tea a day has demonstrated the ability to decrease the initiation and the progression of cancer. More excitingly, green tea has demonstrated the ability to regress established papillomas, which are precursors to tumors. However, according to Hasan Mukhtar, a well-known researcher in the field of green tea polyphenols, "Decaffeinated green tea is not as effective against skin cancer as the caffeine rich variety." Green tea may reduce the risk of skin cancer in people who are exposed to solar ultraviolet radiation.

The American Institute for Cancer Research has collected data on green tea consumption and cancer rates all over the world. They have concluded that green tea may possibly reduce the risk of stomach cancer.

GUAVAS

Guavas are fragrant tropical fruit. These oval, almost pear-shaped fruits turn from green to yellow when ripe. The fruit is ready to eat when it yields to slight pressure. The flesh of guavas owes its red color to its high concentration of lycopene. Guavas are also good sources of ascorbic acid, the plant form of vitamin C. Guavas can be eaten out of hand or mixed into a fruit salad. The skin of the fruit is edible. Puréed guava can be used as a spread for bread.

When people in India with high blood pressure ate four to eight guavas a day, their blood pressure, both systolic and diastolic (the upper and lower numbers), fell by eight points. They also experienced a drop in cholesterol by 8 to 10 percent.

HAZELNUTS. *See* Nuts and Seeds.

HORSERADISH. *See* Radishes.

JERUSALEM ARTICHOKES

The Jerusalem artichoke is a member of the sunflower family and closely resembles sunflowers. They have edible, tuberous, underground stems. They come in many shapes, but basically two types predominate—the whitish, round Western sunchoke and the elongated red Jerusalem artichoke. They need to be scrubbed well to rid them of clinging grit. They are available nearly year-round and can be eaten whole, steamed or raw, or sliced into a salad. They are an excellent addition to soups and stir-fries. Jerusalem artichokes are notable for their high content of fructooligosaccharides, which may be useful in helping to regulate the growth of bacteria in the colon and have the ability to keep blood glucose and insulin levels in check.

A handy way to add Jerusalem artichokes to the diet is by using Jerusalem artichoke pasta. This pasta, which combines semolina flour with Jerusalem artichokes, is made by the DeBoles company and comes in a variety of shapes. It's a little less gummy than ordinary pasta but is every bit as satisfying.

KALE

Kale is a superhero vegetable. If you can develop a liking for its slightly bitter taste, this leafy green will pay you back with a truckload of nutrients. It can be found in a variety of colors, but the most commonly found is the deep-green variety. It is among the fruits and vegetables with the highest known antioxidant capacity with about 1,800 ORAC units. Being a cruciferous vegetable, kale provides the phytochemicals sulforaphane, dithiolethione, and isothiocynate, and the precursors to indole-3-carbinol. It is also a good source of lutein, zeaxanthin, and quercetin and a significant source of the phytonutrients calcium, beta-carotene, and ascorbic acid. Fresh kale is most plentiful and least expensive in the winter months. It can be a lifesaver in meager times because even in the deepest winter, you can still harvest kale from the garden. It also is available frozen and canned in the supermarket.

KUDZU

Kudzu (or kuzu) is an arrowroot starch made from the plant of the same name. The kudzu plant is one of the richest documented sources of the isoflavones genistein and daidzein. Kudzu is a vine that grows wildly in the southern parts of the United States. The kudzu plant is being investigated as a treatment for alcoholism due to its ability to affect alcohol metabolism with its large quantity of daidzin, a compound closely related to the isoflavone daidzein. Most of the kudzu sold in the United States is imported from Asia. Kudzu can be used to make puddings and thicken gravies. It has been used as a remedy in Asia for centuries and is essential in macrobiotic cooking.

According to research available on the isoflavone content of various plants, one tablespoon of kudzu leaves should provide approximately the equivalent amount of the isoflavone genistein as one cup of tofu, a food known for being rich in isoflavones, and about fifteen times more daidzein. The problem is that the kudzu plant is rubbery and wholly unappealing as a food, and the starch extracted from the kudzu plant, which is more appealing and commonly used in cooking, has never been analyzed for its phytochemical content. Should the same high genistein and daidzein content found in the kudzu plant extend to the starch, kudzu will be held in high esteem. If the levels of isoflavones detected in the plant are consistent with the levels found in the starch of the plant, only a small amount of kudzu starch will be needed to achieve the desired level of isoflavones necessary to obtain the health benefits associated with the Asian diet.

LEEKS

Leeks are members of the onion family that look like very large scallions. Leeks contain the phytochemical diallyl sulfide, which may prevent stomach cancer by increasing the production of the enzyme glutathione-S-transferase in the stomach. The green part of the leek is also a minor source of the phytochemicals lutein and zeaxanthin, which might help prevent macular degeneration. Leeks also act as a diuretic, promoting the excretion of fluids from the body. They are sold in the produce section of the market. They're often used as one of many ingredients in soup, but they are delicious vegetables and hold their own when served as a side dish.

LEMONS. *See* Citrus Fruits.

LENTILS. *See* Beans.

LICORICE

Licorice is a perennial herb whose roots are cultivated for their sweet juice extract and for medicinal purposes. It is at the top of the pyramid of foods that the National Institutes of Health are investigating for their anticancer activity. Licorice contains flavonoids, coumarins, and phenols. Glycyrrhiza, one of the main phytochemicals found in the extract of the root, may counteract the action of many prescription diuretics, so it should not be used while taking diuretics. Approximately 100 grams of licorice enhances sodium reabsorption and water retention and complicates therapy for high blood pressure, including diuretic medicines.

LIMES. *See* Citrus Fruits.

MANGOES

Mangoes are luscious, tropical, orange-fleshed fruit that are good sources of fiber, beta-carotene, and ascorbic acid. A cup of mango confers one-tenth of a day's supply of fiber and three-quarters of the requirement of ascorbic acid and beta-carotene. The outer skin turns from green to reddish-yellow when ripe, and the flesh yields when pressed with the finger. Mangoes are sold fresh or jarred as chutneys. Puréed mango can be frozen. To eat a fresh mango, make a long, deep slice with a sharp knife along the length of the fruit until you hit the pit, and cut a wedge. Peel the skin back and discard it. Enjoy!

MISO. *See* Soy Foods.

MUSHROOMS, SHIITAKE

Shiitake mushrooms are significant sources of the phytochemicals eritadenine and lentinan; however, in large doses, raw shiitake mushrooms have been known to cause skin rashes and a feeling of chest heaviness in some people. The incidence of side effects appears to be positively correlated with the amount of shiitake mushrooms eaten, so caution should be exercised with use of shiitake mushrooms. Mushrooms should be cooked; allergic reactions are more likely to result from ingestion of the raw product.

MUSTARD GREENS

Mustard greens are cruciferous vegetables that provide sulforaphane, indole-3-carbinol, dithiolethione, isothiocynate, lutein, and zeaxanthin. In addition, mustard greens are an excellent source of the phytonutrient ascorbic acid. Mustard greens are sold fresh in the produce section of some markets and also can be purchased frozen. Peak months are December through February. In some areas, they are available fresh year-round. Look for fresh young crisp leaves with a deep-green color.

NUTS AND SEEDS

Nuts and seeds are frequently grouped together for the purpose of nutritional discussion because they have similar nutrient profiles. Both are good sources of protein and are named as alternate choices to meat and poultry in the U.S. Food Guide Pyramid. Additionally, both nuts and seeds contain substantial amounts of fat.

The types of fat that predominate in most nuts and seeds are the monounsaturated and polyunsaturated fats, so they are not thought to contribute to heart disease; in fact, they may help prevent it. Two very large clinical trials seem to support this finding. The Nurses' Health Study, which examined the diets and tracked the health states of tens of thousands of female nurses over several years, determined that those who ate more than five ounces of nuts a week had one-third fewer heart attacks than women who seldom or never ate nuts. Similar findings were found among men in the Physicians' Health Study, which examined the health of male doctors. Any type of nuts or nut butter will do. That translates into a small airline bag of nuts or about one-third of the average-size jar of peanut butter. Remember, though, that although eating nuts appears to confer health benefits, nuts are still high in fat, even if they are beneficial fats, and if eaten in excess they can contribute to obesity.

The phytochemicals of note that have been isolated from nuts and seeds are the phytosterols beta-sitosterol, campesterol, and stigmasterol. Phytosterols are plant sterols found in plant cell walls. They are similar in structure to human sterols, which are major constituents of cell membranes in humans and are needed for the creation of reproductive hormones. Pumpkinseeds are very rich in phytosterols, followed by Brazil nuts, sunflower seeds, peanuts, almonds, sesame seeds, soybeans, flaxseeds, and walnuts. Nuts and seeds are also good sources of fiber.

A peanut butter sandwich might make a good lunch choice for a man who has been diagnosed with benign hyperplasia of the prostate gland. One researcher found that 60 milligrams of beta-sitosterol, the amount found in a little more than an ounce of peanuts, significantly helped to reduce the symptoms of benign hyperplasia of the prostate and improved urinary flow.

OAT BRAN

Oat bran is the outermost part of the whole oat or oatmeal kernel. It is removed from the oat kernel through mechanical processing. The

Food and Drug Administration (FDA) recently approved for oat bran and oatmeal the first food-specific health claim, which reads, "Soluble fiber from oatmeal as part of a low saturated fat, low cholesterol diet may reduce the risk of heart disease." One-half cup of fiber-rich oat bran a day has demonstrated the ability to lower total cholesterol by an average of 25 mg/dl (milligrams per deciliter) in a variety of populations. Soluble fiber is well known for its ability to prevent the absorption of cholesterol metabolites in the digestive tract.

OLIVES

Olives are among the most ancient of all foods. There are repeated references to olives in the Bible, and, according to Greek mythology, the olive tree was the gift that Athena brought to the city of Athens as it was being created. In gratitude for her offering, the city carries her name. Olives and the olive oil that is pressed from them are among the richest sources of monounsaturated fatty acid. The oil expressed from olives, whether it be extra virgin olive oil, known for its distinct flavor and deep-green color, or common olive oil, the percentage of monounsaturated fatty acids remains constant at 77 percent. Olives and their oils also contain tocopherols, flavonoids, anthocyanins, sterols, and phenols. Extra virgin olive oil has the highest content of polyphenols and thus delivers the most antioxidant activity. Monounsaturated fatty acids appear to protect good cholesterol, decrease bad cholesterol levels, and decrease total blood cholesterol levels. Diets rich in monounsaturated fatty acids also may be linked to a lowered risk of diabetes.

In the area of the world that surrounds the Mediterranean Sea, olive trees have been cultivated since about 3000 B.C. In ancient times, as well as now, olive oil was the main source of dietary fat in the diets of people in areas where cattle could not survive and dairy products were scarce. From studying the health of those who populate the Mediterranean region, researchers have observed lower rates of heart disease and cancer. This protection from disease is thought to come from their diets, which are high in the monounsaturated fats found in olives.

ONIONS

Onions are members of the allium family, which includes leeks, garlic, chives, and shallots. Onions come in a wide variety of sizes and colors. Diallyl sulfide is the phytochemical compound that appears to be responsible for this group's anticancer abilities. Diallyl sulfide increases the production of the enzyme glutathione-S-transferase, which protects against cancer, in the stomach. In Vidalia, Georgia, home of the Vidalia onion, onions are consumed in large quantities. The death rate from stomach cancer is 50 percent lower there than the national mortality rate from stomach cancer. Red and yellow onions are also sources of the flavonoid phytochemical quercetin, which inhibits both cancer and heart disease. Onions are available fresh, frozen, and dried.

ORANGES. *See* Citrus Fruits.

PAPAYAS

Papayas are tropical fruits that are the sole source of the protein-digesting enzyme papain. They also contain some beta-carotene and ascorbic acid. Papain is useful for improving digestion.

PARSLEY

Parsley is a member of the umbelliferous group of plants, whose leaves are graceful and umbrellalike. There are over thirty varieties of parsley. The word "parsley" is from the ancient Greek, meaning celery growing among the rocks. It is hardy and easy to grow and about as useful and as versatile as one can expect a plant to be. It is notable for its rich nutrient and phytochemical content. The plant contains some ascorbic acid, coumarin, alpha-tocopherol, beta-carotene, carveol, caffeic acid, chlorogenic acid, fiber, geraniol, kaempferol, limonene, quercetin, and selenium. It is rich in lutein. Parsley seeds also contain phthalide.

PARSNIPS

Parsnips are root vegetables similar in appearance to carrots. Like carrots, they are members of the umbelliferous family of vegetables, which are distinguished by the umbrellalike greenery that grows from their tops. Parsnips are among the vegetables being investigated for their anticancer activity and phytochemical content by the National

Institutes of Health. According to Dr. James Duke's Phytochemical and Ethnobotanical Database, parsnip roots contain ascorbic acid, fiber, kaempferol, and limonene. The leaf of the plant also contains quercetin.

PEACHES

What could be more welcome than the first peach of summer? Fresh peaches are fair sources of beta-carotene and good sources of ascorbic acid and fiber. A cup of sliced peaches provides one-tenth of the daily requirement of vitamin A and fiber. Yellow peaches are probably richer sources of beta-carotene than the white variety.

PEANUTS. *See* Nuts and Seeds.

PEARS

In northeast America, autumn is synonymous with the arrival of a new crop of pears. Their colors rival the glory of fall leaves. Whether you choose a green Bartlett, which ripens to a golden yellow, or a red Seckle pear, your pear will provide you with a healthy dose of pectin, the soluble fiber that helps lower blood cholesterol levels.

PEAS

Here's some good news for those who wince at the mere mention of spinach. Green peas are a minor source of those valuable phytochemicals lutein and zeaxanthin that are found so abundantly in leafy green vegetables like spinach. They are also a fair source of the phytonutrients folic acid, beta-carotene, and ascorbic acid—the plant form of vitamin C.

PEPPERS, RED

Red peppers contain the carotenoid lutein, which is a yellow pigment associated with a lower rate of age-related macular degeneration, the leading cause of blindness in the United States after age sixty-five. Peppers also have demonstrated antioxidant activity in studies. Fresh red peppers are also good sources of ascorbic acid and beta-carotene. Hot red peppers contain the phytochemical capsaicin, which suppresses cholesterol formation in the liver and is used topically to treat inflammation. Red peppers are sold fresh in the produce section, sliced and frozen for stir-fries, and dried as flakes.

PINEAPPLES

Pineapples are tropical fruits that are fair sources of ascorbic acid and beta-carotene; however, they are very rich in the protein-digesting enzyme bromelain. Bromelain taken from the fruit of the pineapple has the ability to increase the action of antibiotics when taken simultaneously with them. Bromelain taken from pineapple stems is used therapeutically for its modulation of blood coagulation due to its inhibition of platelet aggregation, anti-inflammatory action, antitumor action, enhancement of the healing process, cardiovascular and circulatory improvement, digestive assistance, and ability to dissolve excess mucus.

PISTACHIOS. *See* Nuts and Seeds.

PLUMS

Plums have significant antioxidant properties. They contain the flavonoids quercetin and anthocyanin, which impart the rich reddish-purple hue of their skins. Plums provide a small amount of ascorbic acid and some beta-carotene to the diet. Choose plums with tight skins that yield to slight pressure applied by the thumb. They are most available in the summer months but can be eaten dried as prunes year-round.

POMEGRANATES

Pomegranates are leathery-skinned, red, ball-shaped fruits that are sold in the markets in the autumn. They are among the few fruits that contains phytoestrogens, although in a relatively small amount. If you peel away the skin of the pomegranate, you will see that it contains many tiny whole seeds that are packed in clusters and compartmentalized between membranes. The seeds are actually tiny whole fruits, which actually contain estrone (a phytoestrogen). Preparing a pomegranate can be tricky. The yellow-white membrane that separates the fruit into clusters is bitter, which makes juicing the pomegranate in the conventional fashion impractical. The seeds need to be removed from the casing before they can be juiced or eaten. They are somewhat troublesome to eat, but when you get a good pomegranate, it is worth the trouble. Pomegranate juice is used to produce grenadine syrup.

POTATOES

Potatoes possess both protease inhibitors and flavonoids, in addition to their high vitamin-C content. To maximize phytochemical content whenever possible, prepare and consume potatoes with the skins intact. Yes, unpeeled potatoes can be mashed. Potatoes are sold fresh, frozen as French fries and hash browns, canned, and dried.

PRUNES. *See* Plums.

PUMPKIN. *See* Squashes.

PUMPKINSEEDS. *See* Nuts and Seeds.

PURSLANE

Purslane is a leafy green that grows abundantly in a wide variety of locales. It is denounced as a weed by some people and valued by others. In *Walden, or Life in the Woods,* Henry David Thoreau wrote, "I have made a satisfactory dinner, satisfactory on several accounts, simply off a dish of purslane (*Portulaca oleracea*), which I gathered in my cornfield, boiled, and salted." Thoreau appreciated purslane for its economy and its taste, but even he could not know its true worth. Purslane is one of the few known land sources of the omega-3 fatty acids that fish and flaxseeds are prized for. Purslane is also a source of ascorbic acid and beta-carotene. The end tips can be added easily to a salad to vary and intensify the salad's phytochemical content. Chopped purslane can be added to a rice casserole, and the fleshy stem can be pickled in brine like a cucumber.

RADISHES

Radishes and their cousin horseradish contain kaempferol, a flavonoid phytochemical with anticancer properties, as well as protease inhibitors. Typically, those radishes found in the produce section of the supermarket are round and pinkish-red in color. They are often included in crudité platters for dipping in a creamy sauce. Rarely are they used as a dinner vegetable, but according to Barry Ballister, who operated a fruit and vegetable stand in Woodstock, New York, for many years, radishes can even be cooked and served warm. In addition to the standard globe-shaped radishes, there are also long, white Japanese radishes and rose-colored Chinese radishes that are used extensively in Asia. They have a creamy texture and a taste similar to turnips when cooked. Horseradish, which has a tangy taste and can be used with milder foods, is sold most frequently in the dairy case in bottles but is sometimes available fresh in the produce section.

RAISINS. *See* Grapes.

RASPBERRIES. *See* Berries.

RICE. *See* Whole Grains.

ROMAINE LETTUCE

Like other green, leafy vegetables, romaine lettuce is a source of lutein and zeaxanthin, the phytochemicals that form the yellow pigment in the macula of the eyes. Romaine is also a fair source of beta-carotene. It is the most nutritionally dense of all the lettuces. Romaine lettuce is available all year fresh in the produce section of the supermarket.

ROSEMARY

The herb rosemary is known as the herb of remembrance. This romantic association may have some scientific basis. There have been three anti-Alzheimer's phytochemicals isolated from this herb—fenchon, thymol, and carvacrol. In addition, rosemary contains the phytochemical carnosol, which appears to have anticancer activity. Rosemary is available fresh in bunches in the produce section or dried in the spice section of the supermarket.

RUTABAGAS

Rutabagas are root vegetables that belong to the mustard family and are closely related to the cabbage family. They come in yellow and white varieties, but the yellow is more widely eaten. Rutabagas contain the phytochemicals indoles and isothiocynates and are fairly good sources of beta-carotene and ascorbic acid. Rutabagas, also called Swedish turnips, are cold-weather crops and have sustained families through wars and famines. They were staples that helped European families survive the harsh winters of World War II when food was scarce.

RYE. *See* Whole Grains.

SCALLIONS

Scallions are actually young onions picked before the bulb develops and are sometimes called green onions. They contain the phytochemical diallyl sulfide, which is known to increase glutathione-S-transferase activity in the stomach. Scallions also contain some beta-carotene and a fair amount of lutein and zeaxanthin.

SHALLOTS

Shallots are small copper-colored bulbs that are members of the allium family. They are often thought of as a combination of an onion and garlic. If you would consider garlic as robust and earthy, then shallots are delicate and elegant. They are used frequently in French cuisine. Shallots are a source of fructooligosaccharides, the fiber that helps to promote beneficial bacteria in the colon. Shallots also contain diallyl sulfide, which predominates in the onion family and is known to increase glutathione-S-transferase activity in the stomach. They are available year-round and are found in the supermarket near the onions and garlic.

Soy Foods

Soybeans are legumes, and technically they should be included as part of the legume section. But since soybeans are processed into so many foods and are so phytochemically dense, they need to be set apart in a section of their own to describe the multitude of ways they can be used to boost the phytochemical content of the diet.

In Asia, soy foods make up a large part of the diet, and people display lower rates of the chronic degenerative diseases that plague Americans. Fortunately, soy foods are beginning to take a foothold in the American diet and are gaining respect for their rich supply of phytochemicals, particularly isoflavones.

Soy foods contain carotenoids, coumarin, fiber, isoflavones, lignans, phenols, phytate, phytosterols, protease inhibitors, and saponins. Once soybeans are processed into other foods, their phytochemical content changes. Some soy foods are richer sources of phytochemicals than are others. Table 4.1 shows the isoflavone content of selected soy foods to help you quantify the amount of isoflavones that different soy foods deliver.

Green Soybeans

Green vegetable soybeans, which are also called edamame (eh-DAM-uh-may), are harvested just prior to their maturity. Cooked and lightly salted, these little green beans are a popular snack in China. The beans, which are often sold in the freezer section of Asian food markets or natural food stores, come preboiled and are made edible in just minutes after reviving them in boiling or steaming water. Slipping the beans out of the pod is part of the fun of eating them. These beans should be stored in the freezer. Fresh soybeans purchased still in the pod should be cooked and stored in the refrigerator.

Miso

Miso is a fermented paste made from soybeans, salt, water, and a cultured grain starter. It is used to make soup and flavor foods. It can be thought of as the Asian equivalent to bouillon, as it is generally kept on hand to add flavor to soups and broths, just as bouillon is often kept on hand in American homes. Miso comes in a variety of flavors and colors. Tastes depend upon the vessel used for fermentation and the length of fermentation time. White miso is milder than the darker varieties. The isoflavones genistein and daidzein have been detected in high quantities in miso. It is available in natural foods stores in the refrigerated section. Miso can be kept in the refrigerator for up to one year.

To make miso soup, dissolve one-half to two-thirds tablespoon of miso in a cup of hot water. In Asian restaurants, this soup is served topped with chopped scallions and a few cubes of tofu.

Soy Flour

Soy flour is made from roasted soybeans that have been ground into a fine powder. It's available in two varieties. Natural soy flour contains the natural oil of the soybean and needs to be stored in the refrigerator. Defatted soy flour is a more concentrated source of protein and needs no refrigeration; however, untreated soy flour is a better source of phytochemicals. Soy flour can be used as a substitute for part of the

Table 4.1. Approximate Isoflavone Content of Selected Soy Foods

Soy Food	Total Isoflavones
Miso (½ cup)	40 mg
Soy flour (½ cup)	50 mg
Soybeans (cooked, ½ cup)	35 mg
Soymilk (½ cup)	40 mg
Tempeh (½ cup)	40 mg
Textured soy protein (cooked, ½ cup)	35 mg
Tofu (½ cup)	40 mg

wheat flour in recipes. For each cup of flour called for, use one-quarter cup soy flour and three-quarters cup wheat flour. Soy flour is gluten free. When using soy flour as a thickener, twice as much is needed as wheat flour to achieve the same results.

Soy Oil

Eighty-five percent of the fat content of the oil expressed from soybeans is unsaturated fat, and about 45 percent of its fatty-acid content is monounsaturated fat, which makes soy oil a factor in maintaining heart health. Soy oil is also a good source of phytosterols—327 milligrams of phytosterols are found in 3.5 ounces of unrefined soy oil. It is also a good source of alpha-tocopherol.

Soy Protein

When protein is removed from defatted soy flakes, the result is called soy protein isolate, the most highly refined soy protein. It contains 92 percent soy protein—the greatest amount of protein of all soy products. Soy protein isolates and concentrates are significant sources of isoflavones only if they have not undergone alcohol processing. Soy protein isolates and concentrates are used to create a variety of products found in natural food stores. Check with the manufacturer of the product that you are using to determine if it has undergone alcohol processing to determine its isoflavone content.

Texturized soy protein usually refers to products make from textured soy flour, although the term also can be applied to textured soy protein concentrates. Texturized soy protein is an excellent source of isoflavones; in fact, it is second only to soybeans in its isoflavone content. It is a dry, granulated product that is usually rehydrated before it is included in recipes. Sometimes, it is marketed under the term "textured vegetable protein" (TVP). It serves as the base for many prepackaged veggie burgers. Fortunately, it is also easy to use in your own kitchen. It can be mixed with ground meat to extend it, or it can be used by itself. It is sold dried in natural food stores. It can be used in the same way ground meat is used to make chili, burgers, tacos, and spaghetti sauce.

Soy Sauce

Soy sauce is a dark brown, salty-tasting liquid made from fermented soybeans. There are three types of soy souce: shoyu, tamari, and teriyaki. Shoyu is a blend of soybeans and wheat. Tamari is made from only soybeans and is a by-product of miso production. Teriyaki is often thicker than shoyu and tamari and contains additional sugar, vinegar, and spices. The commercial soy sauce bought in American supermarkets often contains no soy at all and are often made with artificial colorings and flavorings. Though there are no isoflavones found in soy sauce, the fermenting process used to create these sauces adds nutrients. The bacteria used for fermentation synthesize additional enzymes and vitamins.

Soymilk

Soymilk is made by soaking, grinding, and then straining soybeans into a liquid solution. It is lactose free and comes in an assortment of flavors and fat contents. Soymilk is easier to accept as a substitution for cow's milk if the fat content of the soymilk you choose is at least equal to the fat content of the cow's milk you now use. Soymilk varies widely in its soy-protein content. Twenty-five milligrams of soy protein per day have been shown to have a cholesterol-lowering effect. If you are using soymilk for this reason, check the label to ensure that your soymilk provides at least 25 milligrams of soy protein per serving. Soymilk is one of the easiest ways to work soy into the American diet. It can be used successfully in recipes where cow's milk is normally used, such as puddings, gravies, cereals, and milk shakes. Some soymilks are fortified with vitamins and minerals to mimic cow's milk in nutrient content. Using soymilk as an ingredient in everyday foods that require the inclusion of milk is an acceptable way to introduce soymilk to the diet of the more skeptical eater.

Tempeh

Tempeh is a fermented soy product that is a staple in the Indonesian diet. Tempeh is notable for its vitamin B_{12} content, as this vitamin is seldom available from plant sources. Tempeh is also a good source of isoflavone phytochemicals. It has a meaty texture and can be used in stir-fries and can hold up well enough to be used on the grill.

Tofu

Tofu is soybean curd made through a process similar to the one used in the manufacture of cheese. It is sold in supermarkets, natural food stores, and Asian markets packaged in a water-filled container. It is available in silken and firm textures. It needs to be kept refrigerated and will stay fresh in the refrigerator about five days after it's opened, if the water bath is changed daily. The firm-textured tofu is more suitable for stir-frying and other recipes in which the tofu must be chopped or sliced, whereas the silken tofu lends itself better to making smoother creations like shakes and puddings.

Tofu has been recognized for its phytochemical content—it contains soy protein, isoflavones, phytosterols, and protease inhibitors—as well as its calcium content. But not all tofu is created equal with regard to calcium. Only tofu that has been set with calcium will have significant calcium content. Consult the label to see if calcium is among the ingredients. One-half cup of calcium-set tofu has 258 milligrams of calcium, 80 of which are absorbable by the body. Eight ounces of milk has 300 milligrams of calcium, 96 of which are absorbable.

SPINACH

Spinach is available fresh, frozen, and canned. It is a very rich source of lutein, zeaxanthin, and beta-carotene. It is also a source of protease inhibitors and calcium; however, due to the high content of oxalates (compounds that compete with calcium for absorption) in spinach, the calcium present in spinach is largely unavailable for absorption. Spinach is a high-antioxidant food. When tested with several other vegetables for its oxygen radical absorbance capacity, it beat out all of the other vegetables but kale!

SQUASHES

There are many varieties of squash, ranging from the delicate spaghetti squash of summer to the sturdy winter acorn squash. Generally, squashes are rich sources of beta-carotene. Larger quantities of beta-carotene are present in the squashes with the deepest-colored flesh. Pumpkins and butternut squash are excellent sources of beta-carotene, whereas zucchini and spaghetti squash are relatively poor sources. Winter squash is also a good source of fiber. The type of squash that is available in the produce section varies with the season. Squash is available fresh, frozen, and canned.

SUNFLOWER SEEDS. *See* Nuts and Seeds.

SWEET POTATOES

Surprisingly, sweet potatoes are related to neither potatoes nor yams. They actually belong to the morning glory family. Sweet potatoes are root vegetables and are incredibly rich sources of beta-carotene. One cup of sweet potatoes provides 30 milligrams of beta-carotene. The amount of beta-carotene increases when the vegetable is eaten with the skin on. Sweet potatoes are also good sources of alpha-tocopherol, ascorbic acid, and fiber. A fact that might interest people with diabetes is that a serving of sweet potato will increase blood sugar levels less than would an equal serving of white potato, since white potatoes contain more carbohydrate.

SWISS CHARD

Swiss chard is a large leafy green that looks something like a sturdy, deep-green romaine lettuce. Sometimes it has red veins running through it. Swiss chard contains lutein and zeaxanthin. It grows very easily in the garden or terrace pot and can be harvested when small and added to salads.

TEMPEH. *See* Soy Foods.

TOFU. *See* Soy Foods.

TOMATOES

Tomatoes are abundant sources of the powerful antioxidant carotenoid ly-copene and excellent sources of beta-carotene; in fact, they are second only to carrots as sources of beta-carotene. Tomatoes are also sources of the flavonoids quercetin and kaempferol. They are available fresh, dried, canned, and packed in pasteurized boxes. The more concentrated the source of tomato is, the more lycopene is detected. For example, sun-dried tomatoes and tomato paste, from which the water has been removed, have more lycopene than fresh tomatoes and tomato sauce. Heat and oil seem to enhance the availability of lycopene, so canned tomato juice and spaghetti sauce are very good sources of lycopene. Quercetin and kaempferol serve as a plant's protection from ultraviolet light; thus toma-toes grown in greenhouses have less of these phytochemicals than toma-toes grown in the open air, as the glass blocks out the ultraviolet light. Researchers have noted a 34-percent decreased risk of prostate cancer among men who eat two to four servings of tomato products a week.

TURMERIC

Turmeric is a spice that is often used in Southeast Asian cooking. It is also a component of curry powder. Turmeric is an excellent source of the antioxidant compounds curcumin and tumerin.

TURNIPS

Turnips are relatives of cabbage. This root vegetable contains indoles and isothiocynates. They are also fair sources of beta-carotene and ascorbic acid. This cold-weather crop is easy to grow. The above-ground greens are often eaten as well.

WALNUTS. *See* Nuts and Seeds.

WATERCRESS

Watercress is a cruciferous vegetable that is a source of the phyto-chemicals sulforaphane, indole-3-carbinol, dithiolethione, lutein, and zeaxanthin. Watercress is the richest known source of phenyl ethyl isothiocynate (PEITC). PEITC helps protect against cancer by blocking the activation of NNK (4-methyl-nitrosamino)-1-(3-pyridyl)-1-butanone, the most potent cancer-causing substance found in cigarette smoke. In studies, 6 ounces of watercress given to smokers daily appeared to confer a protective effect against cancer.

WATERMELON
Watermelon is a member of the gourd family. It is rich in lycopene. It is also a good source of beta-carotene and vitamin C.

WHEAT. *See* Whole Grains.

WHOLE GRAINS
Whole grains, sometimes referred to as cereal grains, contain carotenoids, coumarins, flavonoids, glucarates, phenols, phytates, and vitamin E. They are rich sources of protease inhibitors and fiber because they come to us with their bran layer in tact. Much of the active phytochemicals are localized in the bran and the germ, so the health benefits of grains are supreme when the whole-grain product is consumed. Whole grains have 200 to 300 times more phytochemicals than refined grains. Whole-wheat flour, historically called graham flour, is a good example of a whole grain. White flour, its poor and distant cousin, has had its bran layer removed by processing and refining. If you seek out whole-grain foods such as those made with whole wheat, brown rice, whole oats, barley, bulghur wheat, and cornmeal, these foods will be rich in bran and will deliver the maximum amount of phytochemicals and phytonutrients.

The fiber found in whole grains is mostly insoluble, which means that it does not break down in water or in your intestines. Insoluble fiber maintains its integrity in the intestines, and its bulky presence speeds up the movement of food through the digestive tract. It provides relief from constipation and diverticulosis and may help to reduce the risk of colon cancer.

ZUCCHINI. *See* Squashes.

So, there you have them—the richest known sources of the most powerful phytochemicals. As you could see from reading this chapter, almost all fruits and vegetables are chock full of beneficial phyto-chemicals. When you consume a diet based primarily on fruits and vegetables, how could you go wrong? Of course, there are times when you cannot always eat the healthiest diet but still want to do as much as possible to remain healthy. What other options are there for obtaining phytochemicals? Chapter 5 will tell you all about phytochemical supplements and how to choose them.

5

Phytochemical Supplements

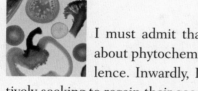 I must admit that I approach the idea of telling you about phytochemical supplements with a bit of ambivalence. Inwardly, I wince when my clients who are actively seeking to regain their good health ask me eagerly, "What should I take?" rather than "What should I eat?" because I am afraid they are seeking a quick cure, and phytochemical supplements will not vault a steady diet of hamburgers and French-fried potatoes into the realm of healthy foods.

Nature packages phytochemicals into whole foods, and if your health-care goal is preventing disease, the best phytochemical delivery system you can use is whole foods. The evidence we have that links certain phytochemicals to disease prevention comes mainly from population-based studies of what people eat and far outweighs the data available from analysis of swallowing isolated phytochemicals. For disease prevention, the sum of phytochemical parts is not worth more than the whole food. In the future, we may come to learn that the true value of phytochemicals comes from the synergy, or interaction, between them rather than their individual activities.

On the other hand, I am glad that phytochemical supplements exist because they allow us to upgrade and fine-tune a less-than-ideal diet. A folic acid supplement can mean the difference between a sick baby and a healthy baby to a woman in her childbearing years, and vitamin E supplements appear to protect against the oxidative damage that leads to heart disease. Phytochemical supplements might provide the perfect intermediary step for those people with a less-than-perfect diet who are trying to gain control over disease.

JUICES

If you have stumbled away from good health and are trying to get it back, you might be considering increasing your intake of certain phytochemicals for their ability to influence the disease process. Sometimes, however, it is not possible to eat enough of the fruits and vegetables needed to maximize your phytochemical intake. Juicing provides a good middle ground between whole foods and packaged phytochemical supplements.

Juicing fresh fruits and vegetables gives you the ability to boost your intake of certain phytochemicals in a package most closely resembling what nature provides. A study that examined the fate of three phytochemicals—beta-carotene, lycopene, and sulforaphane—during the process of juicing determined that juicing delivers about one-half of the important phytochemicals present in the original food. The remainder is discarded with the pulp. Some, however, would argue that getting 50 percent of a nutrient is better than getting none of it.

For certain people, drinking copious amounts of juice may be a cause for concern. Those who are obese and those with type I, type II, or gestational diabetes should limit their fruit juice consumption due to the high sugar content in fruit juices; but for others, fresh juice can offer an alternative way of consuming fruits and vegetables. Check out *Juicing for Life* by Cherie Calbom and Maureen Keane and *The Juice*

Lady's Guide to Juicing for Health by Cherie Calbom for more information about the specifics of juicing.

DRIED FRUIT AND VEGETABLE SUPPLEMENTS

Though ideally we would all like to get our phytochemicals from fresh foods, in reality, this is often difficult for some and virtually impossible for others. To make up for this shortfall, several health-food stores offer dried fruits and vegetables in capsule and powdered forms, often called green foods or whole-food supplements. Sol-Ray offers indole-3-carbinol with their dried cruciferous vegetables. Solgar sells a broccoli extract enhanced with 200 micrograms of additional sulforaphane. This is one way of ensuring that your veggies are replete with at least one phytochemical, but there is no guarantee that any of the other phytochemicals associated with cruciferous vegetables are present.

Taking dessicated vegetables or freeze-dried or crystallized fruit and vegetable juice combinations may be more palatable and more convenient for some people than eating the actual food. It would cost about $1.10 a day to follow the manufacturer's recommended dosages for the dried fruit and vegetable product Greens and More produced by the Solgar Company Earth Source. Considering that a head of broccoli costs approximately $2.00, the cost of supplementation doesn't seem very expensive; but keep in mind that the actual broccoli also provides additional calories for energy, fiber, and some vitamins and minerals that are missing from the supplements.

There is also a large assortment of products referred to as "green foods" in health-foods stores. Nature's Plus makes a product called Green Lightning, which is a whole-food concentrate of young barley plants. Some are powdered to be mixed with water, others are sold in tablet form. They range in price from about $.45 a day to $.70 a day, depending on the brand.

NUTRCEUTICALS

Nutraceuticals are any food or part of a food that provides health benefits, including the prevention and treatment of disease. When circumstances require a dose of phytochemicals that exceeds the amount that can be obtained from food, supplements that supply isolated amounts of phytochemicals, like bromelain or silymarin sold in pills or capsules, are available. Used under the direction of a competent health-care practitioner, these nutraceuticals might offer therapeutic results. Since it would be impossible to obtain the same amount of phytochemicals from food, the phytochemicals are really being used as a pharmaceutical, or pharmafood, and their intake should be monitored by a professional. A health-care professional will know if you are treating a symptom that could be indicative of a potentially dangerous condition. If you desire an integrated approach to health care that involves medicine augmented by the therapeutic use of nutrients and herbs, seek out a physician who works with other health-care professionals who deliver this service.

OILS

Another way to obtain an abundant amount of desired phytochemicals is by using the oil that has been extracted from foods or oil-filled capsules. Garlic supplements are often sold as oil capsules, as are flaxseed supplements. Both of these foods are difficult to ingest in large enough quantities to get therapeutic effects by using the food alone. Oil provides an easy and convenient way to get desired quantities. If you are looking for flaxseed oil, select an organic form, found in the refrigerator case, as flaxseed oil oxidizes quickly, and the cold storage should offer some protection. Use a high-lignan oil for extra lignan content. Spectrum Natural, Inc., is a reputable brand.

Taking flaxseed oil in capsules may be more palatable for some, but you pay a higher price for them. I compared the price of a bottle of Organic Flax Seed Oil that contains sixteen servings of one tablespoon each for $7.69 with General Nutrition Centers's (GNC's) store brand of flaxseed oil capsules—ninety in a bottle for $14.50. You would have to take fourteen capsules to get the amount of alpha-linoleic acid in one tablespoon of the liquid. The liquid flaxseed oil costs $.48 a dose, whereas the capsules cost a whopping $2.00.

DRINK MIXES

Drink mixes made of soy protein can provide approximately the same quantity of the important isoflavones found in the Asian diet and can be taken as part of a meal. They can help boost the isoflavone content of the traditional American diet without requiring drastic meal modifications. The difficulty in recommending their use is that the research data currently available that link isoflavones with decreased symptoms of menopause and lower rates of cancer and cholesterol come from looking at populations that are eating whole foods that contain isoflavones, not ingesting isolated proteins or phytochemicals. Genis Soy makes an isolated soy protein called Ultra Soy. It is a drink powder that you mix with water or juice and is available in a variety of flavors.

CHILDREN'S PHYTOCHEMICAL SUPPLEMENTS

One phytochemical supplement made for children combines vitamins and minerals with 50 milligrams of fruit and vegetable concentrate in a gummy-bear-type candy, marketed under the name Yummi Bears. According to the Center for Science in the Public Interest, "It would take about 90 days worth of supplements to get the equivalent amount of phytochemicals that are in a half cup of vegetables from the daily recommended dose of Yummi Bears." Another chewable child-directed phytochemical supplement is made by Nature's Plus. It is called Kid's Greenz and contains 250 milligrams of a blend of "superfoods." This supplement might provide a more potent dose of phytochemicals than Yummi Bears. Parents should be careful, however, to ensure that they do not rely on supplements for their children's good health. Childhood is a critical time in the growth of a child, and nothing can replace the value of a good, healthy diet.

OTHER SUPPLEMENT FORMS

There are a few other phytochemical supplement forms, depending on what you intend to use them for. Chlorophyll—which, in addition to its use as a supplement, can be used as a mouthwash due to its breath-freshening abilities—can be purchased in liquid form. New Chapter makes a liquid ginger supplement called Ginger Wonder Syrup. Bioflavonoids are sold in capsules and in spray bottles for faster absorption and for those who have problems swallowing pills. Gone are the days when we had to pierce vitamin E gel capsules with a pin to apply the oil topically; the market abounds in vitamin-E-supplemented creams and lotions. One of my favorites is a roll-on vitamin E oil made by Orgene.

COMPARING PRICES

Although supplements might appear to be priced comparably to the foods in which they are present, the food also supplies sustenance, which the supplements lack. The food also supplies a complement of vitamins, minerals, and other phytochemicals.

Beginning in 1999, food supplement manufacturers are required to label bottles with a "Supplements Facts" panel, similar to the "Nutrition Facts" label on packages of foods. The label must clearly state the quantity and type of dietary ingredients present in the bottle. This new labeling system makes it easier to compare products for active ingredients.

Nature's Plus makes a supplement called Ultra Juice, which is made by extracting juice from whole foods and combining it with vitamins and minerals and 2,000 milligrams of a phytochemical cocktail in pill form. This product comes in two varieties: one contains mainly vegetable juice, and the other is a combination of fruits and vegetables. The label states that two pills supply the vitamins, minerals, and phytonutrients of six servings of fruits and vegetables. At about $.52 a day, these supplements could prove to be an alternative for those people who fail to get the recommended five servings of fruits and vegetables daily. But keep in mind that these supplements are missing the fiber, caloric energy, and many of the beneficial phytochemicals that have yet to be discovered.

STORING YOUR PHYTOCHEMICAL SUPPLEMENTS

Phytochemical supplement pills and capsules should be stored with the same care you would give to vitamin and mineral supplements. They are best kept in a dry, dark place at room temperature. A kitchen cupboard works well. Make sure the bottle is marked with an expiration date, and do not use the product after that date. Do not buy products that do not provide you with a freshness date. Chemical structures break down over time, and you will wind up with a different chemical from the one you started out with—perhaps a detrimental one—once the supplement gets old.

Sometimes people transfer supplements to smaller, more manageable bottles, but I find if I do this the small bottles wind up hanging around in suitcases, pocketbooks, and carry-on bags, and I become clueless as to what they are at a later date. For this reason, it is a good idea to keep your supplements in their original containers, or count out the number that will be needed for a journey and return any strays to their original bottles as soon as you return.

OPTIMIZING THE BENEFITS OF PHYTOCHEMICAL SUPPLEMENTS

To enhance their absorption, it is probably best to take oral phytochemical supplements just as you would take vitamin/mineral supplements—at mealtimes, either just prior to or up to twenty minutes after eating. In this way, the phytochemicals will be absorbed with the food, which will increase their absorption, and the body will use them as it would if they came directly from the food. With that in mind, to best ensure optimal utilization of supplements by the body, try to take doses that mimic the amount of phytochemicals found in food. For instance, a cup of cabbage probably has about 100 milligrams of indole-3-carbinol. It's unlikely that you can absorb more than three to four times that amount at any one time. If you're taking higher doses than is available from food, try to divide the dosage over the course of the day.

"How will I know if the phytochemical supplements are working?" you may ask. If you are taking phytochemical supplements to prevent a certain condition and that condition fails to materialize, there is, of course, no way of knowing for sure whether the supplements "worked," or if you would have remained healthy anyway. However, once you begin to realize that you are catching less communicable illness, that you are feeling better overall, and over time that you are living a long life relatively free of degenerative diseases, you will know that it was well worth eating all of your phytochemically rich fruits and vegetables and taking your phytochemical supplements.

If you are taking phytochemical supplements for an existing condition, you will know they are working—you'll have objective proof—when the condition improves. Let's suppose that you are experiencing hot flashes and night sweats as a result of menopause. You begin to include in your diet about 100 milligrams of soy isoflavones daily. You soon notice that your night sweats and hot flashes diminish in frequency and severity. You now have evidence that the phytochemicals are working. The amount of time it takes to experience relief from a certain condition will vary from person to person and disease to disease. Some women have reported almost immediate results from symptoms of menopause with the addition of soy products to their diets, but it will take longer, say, to affect cholesterol levels with the same soy intake.

The Safety of Taking Phytochemical Supplements

For the most part, the taking of phytochemical supplements is safe, since they are merely beneficial compounds taken from the foods we eat everyday. The area of concern may be what the safest proportion is to take the supplements in. It appears from large clinical studies of beta-carotene supplementation that overdosing with one phytochemical may block the uptake of others. Therefore, the safest way to supplement with phytochemicals is with whole-food supplements that contain several phytochemicals that work together. This is also a more economical way of supplementing, as it would cost just slightly more to purchase a whole-food supplement than it would to purchase a singular supplement.

Some may have concerns about the use of products made by less reputable companies who may not include all the ingredients listed on the label. In 1999, the Center for Dietary Supplement Research in Botanicals at the University of California at Los Angeles found that, most often, supplements do contain the ingredients that they advertise. If you are still concerned, make sure you use products from reputable, well-known, or recommended companies, such as Solgar and Twin Labs. If you do experience any adverse side effects, share them with your health-care provider immediately.

Make sure you always work with a health-care provider who is well trained in nutrition when taking your phytochemical supplements. If you question the appropriateness or safety of taking any therapy, not just phytochemical supplements, always consult with your health-care provider.

If you find it difficult to take in the recommended amount of fruits and vegetables in your daily diet, or if there are certain healthful fruits or vegetables that you avoid because you don't like the taste, taking supplemental phytochemicals may help you in your quest for health. But don't use them as a substitute for a healthy diet. They are indeed *supplements to*—not *substitutes for*—a healthy diet. Read on for more ways that phytochemicals can help you achieve optimum health.

6

The Basic Healthy Diet for Disease Prevention

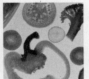 The basic healthy diet is an eating plan that's appropriate for almost all healthy adults. This is an optimal diet for the maintenance of good health. Along the way, I will point out how you can include more phytochemical-rich foods in your basic healthy diet to fight disease and promote optimum health.

When you're changing your diet and your goal is disease prevention, the best results are obtained by moving at your own pace. Don't be impatient with yourself. Dietary changes incorporated into your life gradually as part of an ongoing process rather than as a sudden event will have the most long-lasting effects.

CLIMBING THE FOOD PYRAMID:
BASIC DIET GUIDELINES

The Basic Healthy Diet is based upon the Food Guide Pyramid (see Figure 6.1 below), which was created by the United States Department of Agriculture to give Americans guidelines for the foods they should be eating for optimum health. Following is a list of the food groups that make up the eating plan. For each group, foods that are recommended are specified, as are the foods to avoid. Understand that changing your diet is a process. You and your family will be entering an adjustment period. Small dietary changes are easier to incorporate into your life than a major diet makeover. Little changes made over time can eventually lead to a drastically changed diet.

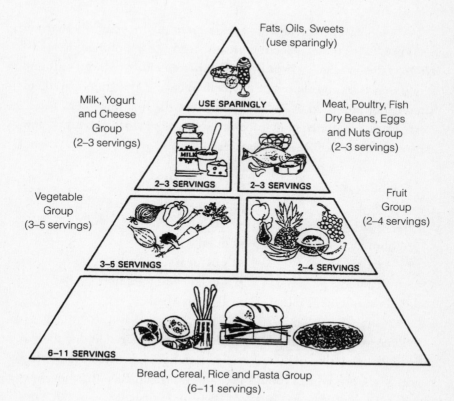

Figure 6.1. Food Guide Pyramid

Grains

The food pyramid calls for six to eleven servings of grain products daily. The grain family includes whole-grain cereals, breads, and pasta products; brown rice; oats; wheat; barley; and corn. A standard serving of grains consists of one slice of bread (approximately 80 calories), or one-half cup of cooked rice, pasta, or cereal. If you eat one-and-one-half cups of pasta, you've had three servings of grains.

Incorporate more whole-grain products into your diet. Experiment with different whole-grain breads and cereals until you find ones that your family agrees upon. There is the potential for waste during this time until you find products that everyone likes. Use the less desirable products to make stuffing, bread crumbs, and croutons so you're not feeling wasteful during the process of finding products your family enjoys.

Whole-grain products will include more phytochemicals than refined products. When selecting breads, read the list of ingredients. If whole grains or whole wheat is the first ingredient listed, you've found a food that is a good source of phytochemicals. If the grain ingredient listed is not preceded by "whole" and is not the first ingredient listed, you're getting a refined grain product with less phytochemicals. Below are some phytochemical-rich breakfast cereals.

- Cheerios
- Muesli
- Nutri-Grain
- Shredded Wheat
- Wheaties
- Wheatena
- Ralston High Fiber

- Granola cereals
- Grape-Nuts
- Bran flakes
- Total
- Oatmeal
- Quaker Multigrain
- Roman Meal

Some cereals that should be eaten only in moderation due to their refined grain content include Basic 4, corn flakes, Frosted Flakes, Just Right, Kix, Corn Pops, Product 19, Puffed Wheat, Rice Krispies, Special K, Cream of Wheat, Cream of Rice, and grits.

Fruits and Vegetables

The food pyramid calls for two to four servings of fruits daily and three to five servings of vegetables daily. A standard serving of fruit or vegetable consists of either one-half cup cooked, fresh, canned, or frozen fruit or vegetable or three-quarters cup of juice. For fresh fruits, a serving size is a fruit about the size of a baseball. For salad greens, a serving size is 1 cup. For dried fruits or vegetables, one-quarter cup fills the requirement for a serving.

All fruits and vegetables contain phytochemicals. Every spoonful of grapefruit might have hundreds of phytochemicals. Some haven't even been discovered yet. Try to stick with locally grown produce in season. Not all countries have the same laws governing the use of harmful pesticides that are enforced in the United States. Or, an even better option is to purchase organic produce to ensure that no harmful pesticides are used at all. Grow your own when possible. Even a small windowsill herb garden can be a rich source of phytochemicals.

Dairy Products

The food pyramid calls for two to three servings daily of dairy products, which include milk, yogurt, and cheese. A standard serving of milk is considered eight ounces of milk or yogurt or one-and-one-half ounces of cheese. One-quarter cup of a wet cheese like cottage cheese also constitutes one dairy serving. One slice of cheese, about the size of a computer disk, equals one serving.

Skim milk or 1-percent-fat products are the most desirable for your health. If your family is not anxious to change, change slowly. If you now drink whole milk, begin mixing the whole milk with 2-percent milk. Then the change down to 2-percent milk won't appear quite as abrupt. Repeat the process to move on to 1-percent milk. Eventually, move on to skim milk. Also, select lower-fat cheeses. Try to use cheese in small amounts like you would use a spice or a condiment to complement the meal rather than as the main focus of the meal.

You may want to consider increasing your intake of nondairy

calcium-rich foods such as broccoli to meet your calcium needs. Did you know that 52.6 percent of the calcium present in broccoli is absorbed and is usable by the body, compared with about 30 percent from dairy products?

Protein-Rich Foods

The Food Guide Pyramid tells us to include two to three servings daily of two to three ounces of protein-rich foods, which include meat, poultry, fish, beans, tofu, eggs, nuts, and nut butters. A standard serving size of chicken, fish, and meat is two to three ounces. Use the palm of your hand as a guide. Your serving should be about that large and no thicker than a deck of cards. A medium egg would also confer a serving of protein. A serving size of cooked beans is one-half cup. Two tablespoons of

A Note on Fish Safety

As an industrial society, we use man-made chemicals and pesticides for processing and growing food. These chemicals are sometimes perfectly safe, but sometimes they are harmful to people. These chemicals eventually seep into our water tables and find their way into lakes, rivers, and streams. The fish that swim in these waters store the chemicals in their fat cells. When we eat these fish, the chemicals are passed on to us.

To cut your risk of food poisoning from fish, the United States Food and Drug Administration cautions people with impaired immunity to avoid raw fish. That includes people with AIDS, cancer, diabetes, cirrhosis of the liver, and compromised gastrointestinal function. To reduce exposure to mercury, keep consumption of swordfish and shark to no more than seven ounces once a week. Pregnant women and other women of childbearing age, children under the age of fifteen, and infants should consume such fish no more than once a month. State cooperative extension offices might have additional warnings about locally caught fish.

peanut butter, one-third cup of nuts, or two tablespoons of seeds constitutes a standard serving size and equals one ounce of protein from meat.

Eat red meat sparingly, if at all. Emphasis should be on beans, tofu, fish, and chicken. Again, try to move away from centering the meal around meat. Purchase and serve small portions of animal foods. Emphasis should be on the plant foods in the meal. Try to look for recipes and ways of preparing meals that include animal foods as a condiment that adds flavor rather than as the focus of the meal.

Fats and Oils

The pyramid advises us to use fats and oils sparingly. We are finding out that some fats are less likely to cause health problems than others. Some fats might even be beneficial to our health, so you should know the differences among the types of fat.

Fat that is found in meat, butter, and cheese is rich in saturated fat. A diet high in saturated fats can lead to clogged arteries, which contributes to heart disease. The American Heart Association advises us to reduce our intake of saturated fat to less than 7 percent of our daily calories. In a 2,000-calorie-a-day diet, 140 calories a day can come from saturated fat. Four 8-ounce glasses of whole milk provide 180 calories from saturated fat, exceeding the allotted amount.

Liquid vegetable and corn oils are rich in polyunsaturated fat. Polyunsaturated fat lowers the LDL (unhealthy) cholesterol but also lowers the HDL or (healthy) cholesterol. Hydrogenated polyunsaturated fats, found in commercially baked goods and margarine, are rich in trans fatty acids and act in a similar fashion as saturated fats to clog the arteries and impede the flow of blood to the heart. If you choose to use margarine, select one packaged in a tub or squeeze bottle rather than a stick; they are lower in trans fatty acids. In addition to adding to the risk of cardiovascular disease, the omega-6 polyunsaturated fats found in vegetable oils appear to stimulate tumor growth in animals. It's best to limit your intake to 10 percent or less of your total calorie intake.

Monounsaturated fats found in olive and canola oils, as well as avocados and nuts, are among the best documented of the heart-healthy fats available. They should constitute about half of your fat intake.

Whenever possible in recipes, substitute olive oil for other fats. Olive oil has centuries of history in the prevention of disease. It has been consumed for centuries in the Mediterranean Sea area where heart disease rates are very low. Canola oil is a relatively new oil that has been genetically engineered to be high in monounsaturated fats. It is about three times higher in the omega-6 fatty acids that can promote cancer growth in animals than olive oil. Canola oil is sometimes preferred over olive oil because its flavor is rather neutral, so it has less effect on the taste of a recipe than olive oil.

Other fats to consider are the omega-3 fatty acids found in fish and flaxseed oil, which are heart-healthy. The taste of fish oil limits its array of uses. The problem with flaxseed oil is that its beneficial chemical structure cannot withstand the heat needed for cooking.

All fats have the same amount of calories. As beneficial as some fats might be for your heart, fats have more calories than any other food, and excess intake can contribute to unwanted pounds, so we are well advised to limit their intake.

Sweets

We are also advised to use sweets sparingly. The United States Department of Agriculture advises us to limit sugar intake to about 32 grams—eight teaspoons—a day for a 2,000-calorie diet. An average cup of fruit yogurt has about six teaspoons of sugar. To make a healthier yogurt, purchase plain low-fat yogurt and add one-half teaspoon of vanilla extract and one teaspoon of maple syrup.

Sugar has many aliases. It is also known as invert sugar, corn sugar, milk sugar, maple sugar, brown sugar, corn syrup, maple syrup, lactose, sucrose, dextrose, fructose, maltose, mannose, glucose, galactose, nutritive sweetener, dextrin, sorghum, honey, turbinado, xylitol, molasses, sorbitol, and mannitol. Table sugar provides calories without any nutrients. That is why you might have heard sugar referred to as having empty calories.

Maple syrup and honey are less processed than refined table sugar and have a minor amount of minerals. Molasses is mineral-rich and has a minimal amount of vitamins as well. These less-processed sugars don't require the body to work as hard at digestion as their more refined cousin, table sugar, does. Therefore, desserts made with less refined sugars are *somewhat* more desirable than those made with refined sugars.

The three things that food manufacturers can manipulate to make commercially prepared food more appealing are salt, fat, and sugar. When they limit or reduce the amount of one of these ingredients, they often increase the amount of another. You, the consumer, have to watch out for this because any of these ingredients has the potential for causing health problems.

If you cut back on fat consumption and use fat-free commercially prepared cakes and cookies that are rich in sugar as a substitute dessert, you risk raising levels of triglycerides (potentially detrimental fats in the blood). People struggling to bring down high cholesterol levels are often drawn to these new products. The problem that arises is that a diet high in simple sugars can raise triglyceride levels and, through this backdoor mechanism, put a person at risk for cardiovascular disease.

SUGGESTED MENUS

What follows is a very basic framework for you to use to devise your own phytochemical-rich diet. Using the information provided within this book about specific diseases, you can create a diet to meet your own needs. Obviously, the portions needed from each group at each meal will vary based on your specific caloric needs.

Breakfast

> ½ cup fruit or juice
> Whole-grain cereal with low-fat milk
> and/or whole-grain bread with a small amount of fat or oil
> (For a healthy adult, approximately 12 eggs a week can be worked into a healthy diet.)

Mid-Morning Snack

Choose one snack from the snack list below.

Lunch

Salad
3–4 ounces of protein (meat/poultry/fish/tofu/beans/nuts)
Whole grains or potatoes
Vegetables
Whole-grain roll

Afternoon Snack

Choose one snack from the snack list below.

Dinner

Salad
Bean or vegetable soup
Sandwich on a whole-grain roll or crackers
(Keep vegetables and beans in mind as you choose a sandwich filling. Try hummus, a veggie burger, or a tabouleh salad.)
Fruit
Beverage

Evening Snack

Choose a snack from the snack list below.

Snack List

Low-fat or fat-free yogurt
Air-popped popcorn
Baked, not fried, whole-grain chips or pretzels
Rice cakes or whole-grain crackers and muffins

Fresh or dried or canned fruits
Vegetables
Fresh vegetable juice
¼ cup nuts, seeds, or nut butters

Notice that I recommended that lunch contain the most animal protein, while dinner includes a substantial amount of vegetable protein. This is because a meal high in carbohydrates, including beans and vegetables, tends to result in an increase in the production of the neurotransmitter serotonin in the brain. This neurotransmitter stimulates drowsiness; thus this effect would be most beneficial for most of us at the end of the day. On the other hand, animal protein like fish, poultry, or meat, if consumed with very little carbohydrates, will induce mental alertness because protein stimulates the creation of dopamine, a neurotransmitter that induces alertness. Most of us could benefit from this effect in the middle of the day. If your day is structured so that you rest in the middle of the day and must be alert in the evenings, switch the dinner and lunch menus.

Over the years, you have probably been inundated with various diet plans, each accompanied by the proclamation that this is the "new" optimal diet. However, research has shown, time and time again, that worldwide, those populations who consume the most fruits, vegetables, and whole grains develop fewer of the diseases that Americans develop most—cardiovascular disease, cancer, and diabetes. So we are faced with a choice—stay with the old diet, based on animal protein and high-fat foods, or switch to a plant-based diet, which has been proven to promote good health and longer lives. Part Two of this book will show you which particular fruits and vegetables you need to incorporate into your diet for the prevention of particular diseases, and Part Three will provide you with some recipes to get you on your way toward following a healthier, plant-based diet.

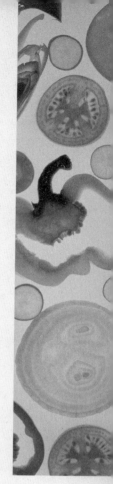

Part Two

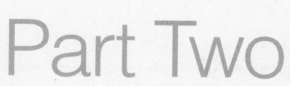

Conditions Treatable or
Preventable with Phytochemicals

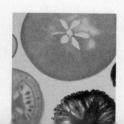

In Part One, you learned all about phytochemicals and in which foods to find them. Now, we are going to put all of that information to work. In Part Two, we will look at the many conditions that can be prevented and perhaps even treated with phytochemicals. Of course, there is no guarantee that a perfect diet will prevent disease; however, study after study shows that those who eat plant-based diets—low in fat, cholesterol, and sodium and high in vitamins, minerals, and phytochemicals—suffer less from chronic, degenerative diseases and live longer, healthier lives.

Of course, if you have or suspect you have a serious medical condition, do not use the information provided in this book to attempt to self-diagnose or self-treat. Your concerns should always be discussed with a health-care practitioner. The information I am giving you is not meant to replace professional advice and treatment, but rather to complement it. Use the information contained herein and become an active participant in the maintenance of your own health.

AGE-RELATED MACULAR DEGENERATION

The macula is a small portion of the retina of the eye that is vital for sharpening visual images. As it degenerates, vision is greatly affected. Age-related macular degeneration is the leading cause of vision loss in persons sixty-five years and older in the United States. As the average life expectancy grows, age-related macular degeneration is increasingly becoming a problem for our aging population. There is no known cure for this devastating eye disease.

There are two types of macular degeneration: dry and wet. In dry macular degeneration, small, yellow deposits of pigment called drusen form beneath the macula of the eye. This is the most commonly occurring of the two types. As the drusen collects, it distorts the central field of vision, causing anything from blurring to blank spots in the visual image. Dry macular degeneration can progress to the more severe wet macular degeneration over a period of time. Wet macular degeneration occurs when abnormal blood vessels form under the macula and the retina. These vessels leak fluid, causing scarring and affecting the patient's central field of vision. Laser surgery may save the balance of the patient's vision. Macular degeneration does not affect peripheral vision.

Phytochemical-Rich Foods to Help Prevent Age-Related Macular Degeneration

Spinach, kale, parsley, collard greens, mustard greens, and other deep-green, leafy vegetables all are excellent sources of the carotenoids lutein and zeaxanthin, the dominant pigments in the macula of the eye. Broccoli is also a good source. Lutein and zeaxanthin have the ability to filter out the wavelength of light called blue light, which might cause oxidative damage to the retina, and therefore protect the blood vessels that supply the macular region of the eye.

In a study done to evaluate the relationship between dietary intakes of carotenoid phytochemicals and the risk of developing age-related macular degeneration, a higher frequency of intake of spinach and collard greens was associated with a substantially lower risk for age-related macular degeneration. The study showed that a daily intake of 6 milligrams of lutein was associated with a 43-percent lower incidence of age-related macular degeneration.

BENIGN HYPERPLASIA OF THE PROSTATE

The prostate is a small male organ about the size of a walnut. It is located beneath the bladder and surrounds the urethra (the tube through which urine exits the bladder and through which semen is ejaculated). The prostate helps in the production of semen. Benign hyperplasia of the prostate is a noncancerous enlargement of the prostate gland, which gradually narrows the opening of the urethra, obstructing the flow of urine. This condition is very common in men over forty years of age of all races and cultures. It may be caused by hormonal changes that occur in men as they age. Hormonal imbalances may lead to the overproduction of the hormone dihydrotestosterone, which causes the prostate to enlarge.

Restoring hormonal balance, thus reducing the body's production of dihydrotestosterone, is helpful in the treatment of this condition. Doctors often use drugs that work on these mechanisms and/or surgery to treat this condition.

Phytochemical-Rich Foods to Help Prevent Benign Hyperplasia of the Prostate Gland

Nuts and seeds are rich sources of the phytosterols beta-sitosterol and stigmasterol. Pumpkinseeds are the best sources of these phytosterols, followed by Brazil nuts, sunflower seeds, peanuts, almonds, sesame seeds, soybeans, flaxseed, and walnuts. Beta-sitosterol appears to prevent the conversion of testosterone into dihydrotestosterone. Large quantities of beta-sitosterol also are found in saw palmetto, which is used as an herbal remedy to treat the symptoms of an enlarged prostate gland.

A clinical study performed in Germany in 1995 on 200 men with benign hyperplasia of the prostate demonstrated that those supplemented with beta-sitosterol, campesterol, and stigmasterol showed significant improvement in symptoms compared with those in the control group who were given a placebo. Sixty milligrams of beta-sitosterol has been shown to reduce the symptoms of benign hyperplasia of the prostate in research studies. This amount can be found in one ounce of most nuts and seeds.

CANCER

Cancer is a disease of the cells' DNA (the part of the cell that carries the genetic information) that evolves in stages. Contrary to popular belief, cancer is not easy to develop. Cancer results after what appears to be a series of biological mishaps. The first stage of cancer is initiation. During this stage, normal cells with normal DNA are attacked by a virus, radiation, or an environmental poison, or the genetic makeup simply goes awry. Once the initiation process is complete, normal cells that usually follow a pattern of division, maturation, and eventual death become mutated. They continue to divide, but they will no longer mature or die. The hallmark of the transformed cancer cell is its immortality.

Scientists believe that an enzyme called telomerase is responsible for the cancer cell's immortality. All cells have telomeres, short strips of DNA, but only cancer cells and sperm cells have telomerase. When a cell is young, it contains a chain of more than 1,000 telomeres. Each time the cell divides, it uses up ten or twenty telomeres from the chain. Eventually, the chain is devoured and the cell loses its ability to reproduce. The chain of telomeres in cancer cells is not exhausted. The length of the chain is thought to be protected by the enzyme telomerase. Scientists believe that telomerase enables the mutated cell to outwit death.

Once the cells have been initiated with cancer, in order for the cancer to advance, it must be exposed to promoters. These are substances that do not change the DNA the way initiators do, but they increase the production of the transformed DNA and stimulate the expression of morphed genes. Promotion must take place repeatedly and over a prolonged period of time for it to stimulate the growth of the mutated cells. The promotion phase may be reversible.

A tumor develops after the initiation and promotion phases have

Can Dietary Changes Affect Cancer That Is Already Present?

The discovery of phytochemicals and their unique abilities to interfere at each stage of cancer fuels the belief that dietary changes can augment traditional therapy in the fight against cancer. Currently, traditional medicine does not offer any hope that dietary changes can be helpful once cancer is diagnosed, but evidence to the contrary exists.

A small research study published in 1993 done at the Tulane School of Public Health showed that the adoption of a macrobiotic diet slowed the progression of prostate cancer in nine men. Of the eighteen men studied, the ones who had adopted the macrobiotic diet lived longer after diagnosis and maintained a better quality of life. This same study compared twenty-three people diagnosed with pancreatic cancer who followed a macrobiotic diet after diagnosis with twenty-three patients with pancreatic cancer who didn't elect to make any dietary changes. The one-year survival rate was 52 percent higher for those who modified their diets than for those who didn't.

A macrobiotic regime is meat- and dairy-free. The bulk of the calories come from whole grains, beans, and land and sea vegetables. While this diet may not be appropriate for everyone, this study provides evidence that dietary changes can be effective after cancer has been diagnosed. Granted, these studies are small, but with the knowledge we are gaining about how phytochemicals work in the body, the increased phytochemical content of the macrobiotic diet could be partially responsible for slowing the progression of cancer. For more information about the macrobiotic diet, read *The Cancer Prevention Diet* by Michio Kushi and Alex Jack.

been active for a long time. A tumor is an overgrowth of cells that are different from the cells around it and serve no apparent purpose. A tumor *in situ* is a localized tumor, meaning that it has not yet spread to other parts of the body. At this point, the tumor is not an immediate threat because the cells at the center of the tumor are too far from the bloodstream to get the nutrients they need to sprout tentacles and grow. Tumors become dangerous when they spread to other parts of the body, a process called metastasis. Tumors begin this process by secreting chemicals that attract specific cells called endothelial cells. These cells develop blood vessels called capillaries, which grow into the tumor. These capillaries act as an "on-ramp," giving the tumor accessibility to send mutated cells throughout the bloodstream. These endothelial cells also pump out molecular messengers called growth factors that stimulate the tumor to divide more rapidly. This process of blood vessel formation is known as "angiogenesis." This is generally a rare event, occurring only during pregnancy, wound healing, and metastasis. Scientists at Harvard are looking into several chemical compounds that interfere with angiogenesis as a way of slowing the growth of cancer to be used as a drug therapy. Soybeans contain phytochemicals that interfere with the process of angiogenesis.

There is no risk involved in adopting a diet high in phytochemicals, and there is some evidence that a high-phytochemical diet can offer cancer patients an opportunity to participate actively in their own treatments.

Phytochemical-Rich Foods That Fight Cancer

For those people who want to make dietary changes to prevent cancer or a recurrence of cancer or to augment current medical treatment of cancer, there are several phytochemical-rich foods that can help.

Cruciferous Vegetables

The phytochemicals from the cruciferous group of vegetables—arugula, broccoli, Brussels sprouts, cabbage, cauliflower, collard greens, kale, kohlrabi, rutabaga, turnips, and watercress—including indole-3-carbinol, dithiolethione, sulforaphane, and benzyl isothiocynate, are considered to be some of the most powerful anticancer substances known. In countries where daily intake of cruciferous vegetables is routine, lower rates of cancer are reported. Try to include at least three to four servings of cruciferous vegetables a week in your diet.

Fresh Produce

Most fresh produce contains chlorogenic acid, which acts as a blocking agent against cancer. Fresh produce is also rich in caffeic and ferulic acids. These acids block the formation of carcinogens and keep the cancer-causing compounds from reacting with the cells necessary to promote and stimulate cancer growth. Yet another phytochemical, quercetin, is found in high concentrations in the outer layers of deeply colored fruits and vegetables. To maximize phytochemical content, eat lots of fresh fruits and vegetables.

Whole Grains

Whole grains contain insoluble fiber, isoprenoids, lignans, vitamin E as alpha-tocopherol, folic acid, and selenium. These are all good reasons to make the shift from refined grain products to whole-grain products.

Beans

All beans, particularly soybeans, contain protease inhibitors, which may slow down tumor growth. They also contain saponins, which interfere with the process by which DNA reproduces and may prevent cancer cells from multiplying. Most beans also possess isoflavones, a phytochemical that blocks the entry of estrogen into the cell, which might slow the progress of hormone-dependent cancers like breast cancer and cancer of the cervix, depending upon a woman's estrogen status. The use of isoflavones in the treatment of hormone-dependent cancers is controversial, since isoflavones have a slight estrogenic ability. There is concern that they may fuel such cancers. There are ongoing studies being conducted to evaluate their effects. Isoflavones from soybeans show promise in slowing the rate of growth of prostate cancer in preliminary studies. To prevent disease, such as cancer, have a serving of beans as your source of protein daily.

Deep-Orange Fruits and Vegetables

Most deep-orange fruits and vegetables, such as carrots, pumpkins, acorn squash, and sweet potatoes, contain beta-carotene, a strong antioxidant that helps to interfere with the initiation of cancer. Our bodies convert beta-carotene to vitamin A. Some other sources of beta-carotene are broccoli and most deep-green, leafy vegetables. The Recommended Dietary Allowance for vitamin A is 800 to 1,000 micrograms of retinol equivalents. A half-cup of beta-carotene-rich food every other day should help you meet this goal.

Onions and Garlic

The entire family of vegetables known as the allium family, which includes onions, leeks, scallions, garlic, chives, and shallots are sources of diallyl sulfide, which increases the activity of an enzyme that protects cells, particularly stomach cells from attack by cancer-causing free radicals. Daily intake of these vegetables should help in the prevention of cancer.

Citrus Fruits

The oil of citrus fruits, which is found in the peel, is rich in limonene. Limonene displays potent antitumor properties during initiation, promotion, and the progression of cancer cells in animal studies. Citrus fruits are also excellent sources of the antioxidant ascorbic acid, the plant form of vitamin C.

Tomatoes

Cooked tomatoes, especially cooked with oil, as in spaghetti sauce, are rich sources of lycopene. It is thought that lycopene may be responsible for protecting against prostate cancer. Men who ate ten or more servings a week of tomato products developed 45 percent fewer prostate cancers than men who ate fewer than two servings weekly in a 1995 study of 45,000 health professionals. This amount also should be useful for you in the prevention of prostate cancer.

Grapes, Berries, and Cherries

Grapes contain reversatrol, which inhibits cancer in its three major stages in laboratory animals. Grapes, as well as berries, also contain ellagic acid, which scavenges carcinogens and may prevent them from altering the DNA of a cell. Cherries contain perillyl alcohol, which has demonstrated chemotherapeutic activity against cancer of the pancreas, breast, and the prostate gland in a variety of animals. Three to four servings a week of grapes, berries, and cherries (when in season) should be included as part of your healthy, cancer-preventive diet.

Green Tea

Green tea contains the powerful phytochemical epigallocatechin-3-gallate (EGCG). It protected against lung and stomach cancer in all three stages of carcinogenesis in a variety of animal studies. Green tea is a potential inhibitor of urokinase—an enzyme that helps cancers to invade cells and spread throughout the body. An intake of four cups of green tea a day has been shown to inhibit the progression of cancer.

Flaxseed

Flaxseed is an extremely rich source of lignans. Lignan bears a structural resemblance to estrogen and can bind to estrogen receptors and inhibit the growth of estrogen-stimulated cancers. In addition, when the omega-3 fatty acid content of flaxseed oil is metabolized, it results in the production of the prostaglandin PG3, a hormonelike substance that enhances the functioning of the immune system.

Phytochemical-Rich Foods That Appear to Be Promising in Fighting Cancer

The following foods are not quite as well studied but appear to have potential in fighting cancer.

Asparagus

Asparagus is a source of saponin, which has shown antitumor activity. Asparagus crude saponins inhibited the growth of human leukemia cells in cell studies. It is not yet known just how much asparagus may be needed to reap such benefits.

Soy Foods

Soy foods also might be helpful in fighting leukemia. The genistein found in soy foods when targeted at leukemia cells in mice was very effective in killing the leukemia cells.

Artichokes

Artichokes are sources of silymarin, a phytochemical that is found in the milk thistle plant. In animal studies, silymarin has demonstrated the ability to work against tumor promotion when tumor growth was stimulated by known carcinogens. Silymarin has previously demonstrated significant activity against liver disease.

Spices

Ginger, turmeric, licorice, rosemary, basil, sage, tarragon, thyme, dill, and caraway contain phytochemicals that have demonstrated the ability to fight cancer.

Other Dietary Recommendations

To prevent cancer, monitor your fat intake. The American Cancer Society recommends a diet where 20 percent of the calories come from fat to prevent cancer.

The bulk of your calories should come from plant foods. Increase your intake of beans, grains, and fresh fruits and vegetables. Five servings of fruits and vegetables a day should serve as a starting point for plant intake. Limit or avoid red meat. Red meat, including pork, causes oxidative damage that can lead to cancer. In addition, meat is a source of arachidonic acid, which has been shown to enhance the spread of cancer, particularly breast cancer. Trade meat meals for fish meals two to three times a week. The omega-3 fatty acids found in fish lead to the production of certain prostaglandins called E3, hormonelike substances that appear to support the immune system.

Use skim milk or 1-percent-fat dairy products. You'll be getting the calcium you need with minimal amounts of fat. Use hormone-free poultry and organic produce if possible. Use whole-grain bread and cereal products.

Limit or avoid foods rich in omega-6 polyunsaturated fatty acids and hydrogenated fats. Corn, safflower, and sunflower oils are high in the omega-6 fatty acids that the body uses to create PG2, a prostaglandin that strongly suppresses the immune system. PG2 is found at the site of malignant tumors. Avoid margarine and processed foods made with hydrogenated fats. Rely mainly on olives, olive oil, flaxseed oil, and avocados for adding fat to your diet.

Avoid smoked, barbecued, and fried foods. The smoking, barbecuing, and frying of these foods create carcinogens. They all are positively linked to cancer. Avoid excessive amounts of sugar. Sugar provides empty calories that will take the place of calories that can come from phytochemical-rich foods.

Suggested Lifstyle Changes

Avoid alcohol and tobacco. Both are linked to cancer, and when used together they are more than twice as potent as when used separately. If you are in reasonably good shape, exercise moderately three to four times a week for twenty to thirty minutes. Someone who is physically active is more likely to have a stronger immune system than someone who is sedentary.

Lastly, think positively. If negative thoughts creep in, create a ritual to rid yourself of them. If you can't do this alone, ask a friend, counselor, or spiritual advisor for help. Larry Dossey's book *Prayer Is Good Medicine: How to Reap the Healing Benefits of Prayer* may be helpful.

Suggested Supplements

Take a multivitamin supplement daily, and if it doesn't contain between 50 and 100 international units of vitamin E, take an additional vitamin E supplement to bring your total intake up to 100 international units. The most active form of vitamin E is d-alpha tocopherol. Be careful not to take more vitamins than you need. 1,600 international units or more of vitamin E has been shown to depress immunity. Limit vitamin C intake to less than 2 or 3 grams (2,000 to 3,000 milligrams) and zinc intake to 50 milligrams or less. Larger intakes of these nutrients also have lowered immune response. For the treatment of several types of cancer, many nutrition-oriented health-care practitioners recommend doses of two or more times the above amounts. Do not take amounts exceeding the above doses except under the care and advice of a health-care practitioner.

CANDIDIASIS

Candidiasis is an infection caused by an overgrowth of the yeastlike fungus candida, which normally exists in the human body in a healthy balance. Under healthy circumstances, the growth of the candida fungus is kept under control by normal biological defense mechanisms. When these mechanisms are disrupted, candida can cause disease.

The incidence of candida infection has risen abruptly since the 1940s when antibiotics came into use. Antibiotics kill the helpful, as well as the harmful, bacteria in the human body. The use of oral contraceptives and corticosteroids may be a predisposing factor for candidiasis. A diet high in simple carbohydrates (sugar) also may contribute to the increased prevalence of this disease. People with diabetes and HIV infection are acutely susceptible to yeast infections. Pregnant women also are inclined to display symptoms of candida overgrowth, which can be transmitted to the infant during its passage through the birth canal.

Commonly, the infection can appear in the gastrointestinal tract where symptoms include a chronic bloated feeling, gas, bowel disturbances, and oral thrush (white, mosslike growth on the tongue). When found in the female genitourinary tract, symptoms include itching and discharge. Some people report chronic fatigue, poor memory, and an inability to concentrate. An overgrowth of candida also can cause a body rash sometimes seen in infants. For more information about candidiasis, read *The Yeast Connection* by William G. Crook.

A medical doctor can diagnose candidiasis and will usually prescribe medicine to treat the affected area. Often the medicine works and the symptoms abate, but sometimes there is a chronic recurrence of symptoms that are only temporarily relieved by prescription medicines. In that case, the next step would be to take responsibility for management of your disease by adopting a diet designed to rebalance the flora in the body.

Phytochemical-Rich Foods to Help Fight Candidiasis

Jerusalem artichokes, shallots, garlic, onions, artichokes, and bananas all are good sources of fructooligosaccharides. Fructooligosaccharides (FOS) promote the growth of bifidiobacteria, healthy bacteria that help to restore the normal intestinal flora whose disruption results in infection with candidiasis. See Table 3.3 on page 46 of Part One for foods rich in FOS. Be sure to include these foods in your diet.

Cinnamon contains the phytochemicals eugenol and geraniol, which are noted for their ability to combat candida. Ginger contains the phytochemicals citronellol, geraniol, and myricetin, which all contain anticandida properties. Rosemary contains the phytochemicals carnosol and geraniol. Each is noted for its ability to interfere with the growth of candida.

Other Dietary Recommendations

More than twenty years worth of anecdotal evidence supports the adoption of dietary changes for the relief of chronic candidiasis. The diet is strict and suggests elimination of many commonly consumed foods. The initial stage of adopting the diet often is fraught with confusion because it seems there is nothing to eat. After closer inspection, you will see that there are many foods available to meet the appetite. The payoff for adopting this strict regime is reclaiming your health.

Foods that can be eaten in abundance by those with candidiasis are fresh vegetables, legumes, fish, lean meat, poultry, nuts, and seeds. Acquaint yourself with those vegetables rich in calcium and eat heartily from that group of vegetables. Limit your intake of yeast and mold. Commercially baked bread is made with yeast. Yeast-free bread is available in natural food stores. Ry-Krisp, Wasa, Kavli, or Ryvita crisp breads or other whole-grain crispy breads are fine grain choices, as are rice cakes, taco shells, and tortillas. Nut butters other than peanut butter (which can worsen your condition) spread on rice cakes make great snacks. Wine, vinegar, beer, and other alcoholic drinks also contain yeast. Also avoid mushrooms because they are mold spores.

Eliminate all sugar from your diet. This includes table sugar, honey, maple syrup, barley malt, fructose, and fruit juice concentrate. Sugar provides a medium that encourages the growth of candida. It is apparent that when a glucose-rich formula is introduced into the bloodstream, candidiasis usually follows.

Eliminate fruit juice and dried fruit from your diet and limit fresh fruit intake to one to two servings a day. Select fruits from those rich in FOS. These will help increase the production of good bacteria, which will counter the negative effects of an overgrowth of candida.

Avoid milk and milk products, except for eight ounces of plain yogurt with acidophilus daily. The lactose in milk will act as a sugar medium in which the yeast can grow. The quantity of lactose in yogurt is reduced because it is a cultured product.

Limit your servings of wheat, barley, oats, rye, corn, rice, potatoes, and millet to about one-half cup per meal. Keep the total servings of all grains down to four or five a day. Select only whole grains. Grains are complex carbohydrates and are necessary for normal body functions, but nevertheless they are carbohydrates, and they provide a source of glucose.

Avoid peanuts and peanut butter due to the mold aflatoxin that is found on peanuts; but other nut butters—for example, almond butter or cashew butter—are fine. Avoid pickled, smoked, and dried meat, fish, and poultry. Any foods that are aged, such as sauerkraut, olives, and pickles, all should be avoided, as should fermented foods.

Suggested Supplements

A good yeast-free multivitamin/mineral supplement will ensure you that you are taking in the recommended daily intake of vitamins. If you are not meeting your calcium needs, which vary from 800 to 1,500 milligrams a day depending on the person, take a calcium supplement. Calcium carbonate and calcium citrate malate are both well-absorbed supplements. Look for a calcium supplement that also includes vitamin D, which is also needed to build bones.

Acidophilus is known to help restore the body's flora to its balanced state. Ask your health-care provider to recommend a specific supplement. For more information, see the book *Probiotics: Nature's Internal Healers* by Natasha Trenev.

CARDIOVASCULAR DISEASE

Cardiovascular disease is a collective term for disorders affecting the circulatory system—the heart and the blood vessels. Collectively, cardiovascular disease is the number-one cause of death in the United States. Outside of congenital disorders, most cardiovascular diseases are caused by inadequate blood flow to the heart, usually due to narrowing of the arteries.

Arteriosclerosis is a condition in which the arteries narrow due to hardening and thickening. *Atherosclerosis* is the most common type of arteriosclerosis, in which fatty material accumulates on the vessel wall, hardening and forming a plaque. This condition can lead to a host of other conditions.

Angina is chest pain caused by inadequate oxygen supply to the heart. This is a result of atherosclerosis. Angina may indicate that one is at risk of a heart attack. *Heart attack*, or *myocardial infarction*, occurs when blood flow to the heart is blocked severely or completely. *High blood pressure*, or *hypertension*, also can result from impaired blood flow in the arteries. When the arteries thicken and harden, it is more difficult for the blood to get through them and less can get through at a time, increasing the pressure in the arteries. Any disorder affecting the heart can lead to *heart failure*, a condition in which the heart is unable to pump enough blood to meet the body's needs.

Assessing Your Risk of Developing Cardiovascular Disease

Routine physicals often include a blood test that determines your blood cholesterol level. According to the American Heart Association, you can use this information in a simple formula to help you ascertain if the cholesterol in your bloodstream is building up in your arteries and increasing your chances of developing heart disease. The formula is as follows:

Divide your total cholesterol count (TC) by the level of your high-density-lipoprotein (HDL) cholesterol—the so-called "good" cholesterol, which does not contribute to heart disease and actually helps rid the blood of excess low-density-lipoprotein (LDL), or "bad," cholesterol, which contributes to heart disease. Ideally, this figure should be 3.5 or less. If the figure you arrive at is more than 5.0, fat is probably accumulating in your arteries. If this is the case, you need to make some lifestyle modifications to change that figure. If you follow the guidelines presented to you in this section, you can raise your blood level of HDL cholesterol and lower your total cholesterol level.

If you are concerned about a child's cholesterol count, consult with his or her pediatrician or family doctor before you limit his or her fat intake.

Cholesterol is often a culprit in cardiovascular disease. Cholesterol can deposit in the arterial walls, leading to arteriosclerosis and any of the other conditions just described. It appears that a diet high in animal fat and a sedentary lifestyle can contribute to the likelihood of developing this type of cardiovascular disease.

Phytochemical-Rich Foods to Help Prevent and Fight Cardiovascular Disease

Don't despair. There are changes you can make in your diet to reduce your risk of suffering from cardiovascular disease or to fight it if you currently suffer from it. The following foods are rich in phytochemicals that will help you fight cardiovascular disease.

Oats

Oats and oatmeal are rich in oat bran, one of the first foods approved by the Food and Drug Administration (FDA) to promote a specific health claim. One-half cup of oat bran, which is found in three-quarters of a cup of dry oatmeal, has been shown to be effective in lowering total blood cholesterol when combined with a diet low in saturated fats and cholesterol. The average drop in cholesterol experienced is 25 mg/dl (milligrams per deciliter of blood). One-third cup of oatmeal daily lowers total blood cholesterol levels by 5 mg/dl.

Foods Rich in Monounsaturated Fatty Acids

Olive and canola oil, avocados, and most nuts are rich in monounsaturated fat. Monounsaturated fat decreases total blood cholesterol and LDL cholesterol levels, while protecting and possibly increasing HDL cholesterol, thus lowering the ratio of total cholesterol to HDL cholesterol in the blood. In countries where olive oil is generously used, there is a lower incidence of heart disease than there is in America.

Researchers have recently found that women who eat five or more ounces of nuts a week have one-third fewer heart attacks than women who seldom include nuts and nut butters in their diets. Preliminary information from a study of men suggests that frequent nut consumption may provide similar benefits in men.

The fats in olive and canola oil, avocados, and nuts should be used as substitutes for the more saturated fats found in meats, cheese, and butter, not in addition to these fats. You must keep your total fat-calorie intake at around 30 percent of your total caloric intake.

Garlic

The allicin found in garlic can be helpful in lowering cholesterol. As little as one-half of a garlic clove daily can reduce cholesterol levels by 10 percent. "The beneficial effects obtained from garlic are best obtained from fresh garlic," according to Dr. Eric Bloch, a researcher at the State University of New York at Albany. In addition to lowering cholesterol, garlic, like fish oil, will make blood less sticky and less apt to aggregate around an obstruction in the artery. Avoid raw garlic if you have ulcers or stomach problems. In one study, subjects were given three 300-milligram garlic supplement capsules daily. A 14-percent decrease in LDL-cholesterol levels was achieved in this study. Obtaining phytochemicals through food, however, is the best way to take them in.

Foods Rich in Soluble Fiber

Add dried beans and barley to your diet. These foods have generous amounts of soluble fiber. The fiber will bind to the excess cholesterol in your body and help carry it out. Current recommendations from the American Heart Association call for an intake of 25 to 30 grams of fiber a day. This amount is adequate in the prevention of cardiovascular disease. Beans serve at least a twofold purpose in creating a more healthful diet. In addition to the phytochemicals they provide, legumes are a filling and protein-rich food that can take the place of less healthful foods. Try to include soybeans and soy products in your diet. In studies, 47 grams of soy protein daily has demonstrated the ability to lower LDL blood cholesterol by an average of 13 percent. However, as little as 25 grams a day is sufficient for lowering blood cholesterol levels.

Foods Rich in Folic Acid and Vitamin B6

Folic acid and vitamin B_6 reduce the levels of the amino acid homocysteine in the blood. Homocysteine is believed to increase the risk of heart disease by nourishing blood clots and narrowing blood vessels; by promoting the growth of smooth muscle cells, which also narrows blood vessels; and by damaging the cells that line the arteries. Be sure to eat lots of foods rich in these B vitamins to stave off heart disease. You should take in 400 micrograms of folic acid and 3 milligrams of vitamin B_6 daily. This is about double the current RDA for those vitamins. Current clinical studies indicate a reduced risk of cardiovascular disease in people whose intake of these two B vitamins is at this level. The table below and the one following list some of the most folic-acid- and vitamin-B_6-rich foods.

Pectin-Rich Foods

Foods rich in pectin include apples, pears, citrus fruits, and berries. The pectin in these fruits will form a gel in your intestines that traps cholesterol and carries it out of the body. Eat at least three servings of pectin-rich fruit daily.

Folic-Acid-Rich Foods

Food	Folic Acid per Serving
Apple, fresh (medium)	4 mcg
Brewers yeast (1 tablespoon)	313 mcg
Broccoli (1 cup)	107 mcg
Lentils, cooked (1 cup)	358 mcg
Orange juice (8 ounces)	45 mcg
Pinto beans (1 cup)	137 mcg
Romaine lettuce (1 cup)	76 mcg
Spinach, cooked (1 cup)	262 mcg

Vitamin-B$_6$-Rich Foods

Food	Vitamin B$_6$ per Serving
Baked potato, whole	.70 mg
Baked potato, no skin	.50 mg
Banana (about 7-inch)	.66 mg
Chicken breast, roasted (one-half)	.52 mg
Orange, fresh (1)	.08 mg
Soybeans (1 cup)	.50 mg
Sunflower seeds (¼ cup)	.46 mg
White bread, enriched (1 slice)	Less than .01 mg
Whole-wheat bread (1 slice)	Less than .05 mg

Phytochemical-Rich Foods That Appear to Be Promising in Fighting Cardiovascular Disease

There are a variety of foods that have less research behind them than the foods named above, but the documentation is beginning to mount, and they may be useful dietary additions to consider when developing a diet to fight cardiovascular disease.

Grape Juice

Eight ounces of purple grape juice demonstrated the ability to decrease the clotting potential of blood by 75 percent in seventeen human subjects. It's well documented that both aspirin and red wine have the ability to make blood less sticky. Many doctors prescribe an aspirin a day for their patients; wine appears to keep heart disease a non-issue in France, although saturated-fat intake is high in that country. But both wine and aspirin are contraindicated for some people. So it's good to be aware that an alternative treatment might exist that can be used daily without negative side effects. Like wine, purple grape juice contains flavonoids. Purple grape juice appears to be more potent than white grape juice in the same way that red wine is more potent than white wine when it comes to its ability to make the blood less sticky.

Flaxseeds

Flaxseeds and flaxseed oil are promising additions to the list of foods that fight cardiovascular disease. In one experiment with female volunteers, when 50 grams (1.75 ounces) of raw ground flaxseed was added to the diet, total cholesterol was lowered by 9 percent and total low-density lipoproteins (LDL cholesterol) decreased by 18 percent. Changes in the plasma fat profile of the blood were similar when the source of the flax was 20 grams a day of flaxseed oil.

Red Peppers

By spicing your foods with red pepper, which is used liberally in Mexican cooking, you'll be adding capsicum to your foods. Capsicum suppresses cholesterol formation in the liver.

Shiitake Mushrooms

Shiitake mushrooms, either fresh or dried, contain eritadenine, which promotes tissue uptake of cholesterol. When cholesterol is taken up by the tissues, it is not present in large amounts in the bloodstream to clog arteries. There is a good study showing that patients who ate four ounces of fresh or two ounces of dried shiitake mushrooms had a 10-percent drop in cholesterol levels in one week.

Green Tea

The antioxidants in green tea are 100 times more effective than vitamin C and 25 times more effective than vitamin E at protecting cells from the injury thought to be caused by oxidative damage that can lead to diseases including cardiovascular disease. An investigation of lifestyle habits in Japan revealed that men who drink more than ten cups of green tea daily have lower levels of cholesterol and triglycerides, regardless of age, relative body weight, alcohol consumption, and cigarette-smoking habits. Even at intakes lower than ten cups, green tea consumption was positively associated with lower serum concentrations of fat. Daily consumption of green tea will help you in the fight against cardiovascular disease.

Other Dietary Recommendations

Monitor your fat intake. As Step I of the American Heart Association's (AHA) Diet Plan, the AHA recommends a diet in which 30 percent of the calories come from fat and 10 percent or less calories come from saturated fats that predominate in animal foods. Spread your fat intake throughout your meals and snacks over the course of the day. Keep some fruit and low-fat snacks available to keep you on track after you've consumed your daily fat allowance. After about three to six months of keeping your fat intake down to 30 percent of your calorie intake, have your cholesterol levels checked. If your total cholesterol divided by your HDL cholesterol is not down to 5.0 or less (see "Assessing Your Risk of Developing Cardiovascular Disease" on page 135), it's time to move on to Step II.

If Step I was not effective for you, you're not alone. Keeping fat intake down to 30 percent of total calories may not be enough to reverse the fat buildup that has accumulated in your arteries. You may find that a diet in which only 20 percent of calories are from fat and 7 percent or less are from saturated fat is more effective in achieving these goals. This is Step II of the American Heart Association's Diet Plan. After three to six months on Step II, have your blood redrawn. If the ratio of total cholesterol to HDL cholesterol has still not dipped to 5.0 or below, there still may be a drug-free option for you. Dr. Dean Ornish was able to help his patients reverse cardiovascular disease with diet and lifestyle changes. Try reading his book *Dr. Dean Ornish's Program for Reversing Heart Disease.*

Overall, avoid foods rich in saturated fat. Large amounts of saturated fat are found in red meat, high-fat dairy products, and chocolate. Saturated fat raises total cholesterol and LDL cholesterol. If you find that you cannot eliminate meat from your diet, substitute fish for meat a few times a week. Fish is rich in the omega-3 fatty acids that decrease risk of cardiovascular disease. Vary your fish intake. Women of childbearing age should limit their consumption of shark and swordfish to once a month; of grouper, marlin, and orange roughy to fourteen ounces a week; and tuna to two pounds a week to limit their exposure to mercury. Also avoid foods made with hydrogenated fat. Hydrogenated fats are processed fats that contain trans-fatty acids, polyunsaturated fats that have been engineered to lengthen their shelf life. Unfortunately, these fats act like saturated fat in the body and raise total cholesterol and LDL-cholesterol levels. Hydrogenated fat is found mostly in solid margarine, packaged bakery products, cookies, crackers, cake mixes, and candy.

Recommended Lifestyle Changes

If you smoke, stop. Smoking constricts the blood vessels, thus making it harder for the arteries to carry oxygen to the heart. If you are in reasonably good shape, exercise moderately three to four times a week for twenty to thirty minutes. Research has shown that HDL-cholesterol levels respond positively to increased physical exercise. Additionally, someone who is physically active is more likely to have a stronger immune system than someone who is sedentary is. Keep your alcohol intake down to two drinks or less daily if you are a man and one drink per day if you're a woman. Increased alcohol intake leads to increased triglyceride levels, which are also a risk factor for cardiovascular disease.

Suggested Supplements

Take a multivitamin supplement daily, and if it doesn't contain between 50 and 100 international units of vitamin E, take an extra vitamin E supplement to bring your total intake up to 100 international units. D-alpha tocopherol is the most active vitamin E supplement available. Be careful not to take more vitamins than you need. About 1,600 international units or more of vitamin E has been shown to depress immunity. Limit intake of vitamin C to less than 2 or 3 grams (2,000 to 3,000 milligrams) and zinc intake to 50 milligrams or less. Larger intakes of these nutrients also have been shown to lower immune response.

DIABETES

Diabetes is the name for a group of syndromes characterized by abnormal glucose (blood sugar) levels, caused by a lack of insulin or a decreased sensitivity to the insulin receptors on cells. Glucose is transported in the bloodstream by insulin. I often tell my clients that insulin works as an escort to bring glucose to the cells of the body. Without sufficient insulin, glucose remains in the blood supply and is not brought to the cells. Without glucose to supply them with energy, the bodies' cells revert to starvation mode.

Type I diabetes, or insulin-dependent diabetes, usually starts suddenly in childhood and is believed to be an autoimmune disease, meaning it is the result of the body's immune system going awry and actually attacking its own body. People with type I diabetes have antibodies to the cells of the pancreas, the gland that produces insulin, circulating in their blood.

Type II diabetes usually occurs after the age of forty-five, frequently in overweight people, and ranges in severity from mere insulin resistance to insulin dependence. Occasionally, children are diagnosed with type II diabetes. It frequently can be controlled with diet and exercise. It is diagnosed when two consecutive blood tests taken while fasting reveal that the level of blood sugar is 126 mg/dl (milligrams per deciliter) or higher.

Impaired glucose tolerance (IGT) occurs when the blood glucose level is elevated but not high enough to be diagnosed as diabetes. Impaired glucose tolerance is diagnosed when blood sugar is found to be between 110 and 125 mg/dl while fasting. Some health professionals believe that impaired glucose tolerance is actually type II diabetes in its earliest appearance. They refer to it as borderline diabetes. Sometimes impaired glucose tolerance is a temporary situation. When it is not, people with impaired glucose tolerance are at increased risk for some the same complications as those with apparent diabetes.

Gestational diabetes occurs during pregnancy and generally goes away once the baby is delivered. It is often an indication of an increased risk of developing type II diabetes later in life. If gestational diabetes is not controlled, the fetus can grow to an abnormally large size, and the fetus will be at greater risk for developing such treatable complications as jaundice and breathing difficulties.

The high blood sugar levels that characterize diabetes need to be controlled and kept within normal limits to reduce the long-term complications of chronic high blood sugar—premature cardiovascular disease, kidney disease, and vision problems. In addition, those with diabetes are constantly challenged to keep their blood sugar levels within normal ranges to diminish the immediate symptoms, including extreme thirst, frequent urination, and blurred vision, that come from the abnormal fluctuations of blood sugar that can severely complicate life.

Phytochemical-Rich Foods to Help Fight Diabetes

Although all people who are diagnosed with diabetes should have a diet specially tailored to their lifestyles and eating habits, there are some guidelines for people with diabetes that are generally recognized as useful and some phytochemical-rich foods that appear to offer promise in helping to moderate blood sugar and in reducing some of the complications of diabetes.

Foods Rich in Monounsaturated Fatty Acids

Monounsaturated fatty acids, which are found in large quantities in olives, olive oil, canola oil, and avocados, have a well-documented ability to effect positive change in blood glucose, cholesterol, triglyceride, and insulin levels for some people with diabetes. Sixty to 70 percent of calories can be distributed between carbohydrates and monounsaturated fats. Furthermore, there is no evidence that a diet high in monounsaturated fats will induce weight gain if total calorie intake is controlled.

Whole Grains

Whole-grain breads and cereals contain more vitamin E (alpha-tocopherol) and fiber than their more refined white counterparts do. A slice of whole-wheat bread has about sixteen times as much vitamin E and three times as much fiber as a slice of white bread does. The same is true when you compare brown rice to white rice. If you multiply those figures by the ten or so servings of grains you eat in a day, you can see how you can significantly increase your vitamin E and fiber intake without even taking supplements, just by switching to whole-grain products. Vitamin E has demonstrated the ability to act as a scavenger of free radicals and to decrease the amount of LDL (low-density lipoproteins) that enter and oxidize the arteries, contributing to the premature cardiovascular disease so prevalent in diabetes. Although people with diabetes are not instructed to eat more fiber than other people, it is critically important that they ingest the recommended 25 to 35 grams a day of fiber, which can be found more readily in whole grains than in their refined counterparts.

Legumes

Legumes, including beans, peas, and peanuts, are good sources of fiber. They also contain tyrosine kinase inhibitors. Both phytochemicals help to offset high blood sugar and some of its long-term negative side effects. When beans are digested, their glucose is released slowly into the bloodstream, helping to keep blood sugar relatively level if measured against another carbohydrate source that is comparable in calories.

Recently, scientist have discovered that tyrosine kinase inhibitors that are found in many types of beans in the form of genistein may help impede the premature cardiovascular disease that occurs with diabetes. One of the tests used to measure long-term control of diabetes is called hemoglobin A1C. It is a measure of the amount of a specific type of protein in the blood. Hemoglobin A1C levels are higher in people with uncontrolled blood sugar than in people who have blood sugar with normal range. Hemoglobin A1C proteins have receptors that generate free radicals, potentially dangerous electrons that produce a substance called tissue factor. Increased levels of tissue factor lead to increased coagulation of the blood, which could help to explain why people with diabetes develop cardiovascular disease earlier than other people.

Tyrosine kinase is involved in transmitting signals in the cell. It sends a message from the cell membrane to the control center of the cell to increase the cell's ability to participate in the coagulation of the blood. So it follows that a food that will down-regulate the amount of tissue factor in the blood may help to reduce the early increased coagulation that leads to premature cardiovascular disease that so frequently occurs in people with diabetes.

Deep-Green and Orange Fruits and Vegetables

Carrots, broccoli, and other deep-green and yellow-orange foods rich in beta-carotene also may help to decrease the premature cardiovascular disease that often occurs in people with diabetes by providing a source of antioxidants to quench the free radicals that are created when blood sugars exceed the normal range. These free radicals can damage blood vessels and make blood more apt to coagulate and block its flow to the heart.

Citrus Fruits and Tomatoes

Citrus fruits, tomatoes, and other good sources of ascorbic acid (vitamin C) also can act as antioxidants to help satisfy free radicals in the cell to decrease the potential damage to the vascular system. Vitamin C works with vitamin E to decrease the oxidation of low-density lipoproteins in the blood, which are most apt to contribute to clogging the arteries.

Phytochemical-Rich Foods That Appear to Be Promising in Fighting Diabetes

There are a variety of foods on which less research has been conducted in relation to their effects on diabetes than on the foods named above; however, the documentation is beginning to mount, and these foods might be useful dietary additions to consider when developing a diet to fight diabetes.

Flaxseed

When people with diabetes ate 50 grams (1.75 ounces or two-thirds of a cup) of ground flaxseed as part of a test meal, postmeal blood sugar levels were 27 percent lower than those taken from subjects who ate the same meal without the flaxseed supplement. This leads researchers to conclude that flaxseed may be helpful for decreasing high blood sugar levels in people with diabetes.

Foods Rich in Fructooligosaccharides

Fructooligosaccharides are found in Jerusalem artichokes, onions, bananas, tomatoes, honey, garlic, and wheat. They have demonstrated the ability to increase glucose tolerance. Some studies have shown that fructooligosaccharides, when used in place of another carbohydrate, will produce less of an increase in blood glucose and insulin levels. Some doctors are recommending that diabetic patients who eat pasta change their pasta to one that includes Jerusalem artichoke flour to take advantage of the fructooligosaccharide content of the product.

Other Dietary Recommendations

People with diabetes should eat at least three meals a day at regular intervals to keep their blood sugar levels within normal range. Meals and snacks that combine carbohydrates with proteins or fats will have the longest-lasting effects on blood sugar levels because protein and fat take longer to raise blood sugar than carbohydrates do. Sugar and non-nutritive sweeteners like aspartame, acesulfame, and saccharin can be used but should not be abused. For the most part, avoid large quantities of sweeteners in your diet.

Suggested Lifestyle Changes

Check your blood sugar regularly and strive to keep it within normal range. Tight control of blood sugar will reduce your risk of future complications from diabetes. People with diabetes should engage in regular exercise. Exercise makes insulin more sensitive and helps the body's cells to recognize glucose. Health-care providers will have more specific exercise guidelines for those with type I diabetes. Alcohol consumption should be limited to two drinks or fewer daily and should always be consumed with food.

Suggested Supplements

For a number of people diagnosed with impaired glucose tolerance, supplementation with chromium in the form of chromium picolinate has helped to improve blood sugar levels. The requirement for chromium is related to the degree of glucose intolerance. Two hundred micrograms a day of chromium is adequate to improve glucose levels of those who are mildly glucose intolerant. However, people with more extreme cases of glucose intolerance (diabetes, for example) usually require more than 200 micrograms a day. Daily intake of 8 micrograms per kilogram of body weight was shown to be more effective than 4 micrograms per kilogram of body weight in women with gestational diabetes. To determine how much chromium you will need to reach 8 micrograms per kilogram of body weight, divide your body weight by 2.2, which will convert weight in pounds to weight in kilograms. And then multiply that by 8. This will provide you with 8 micrograms per kilogram of body weight.

If you're over fifty years old, take a simple multivitamin daily, and if it doesn't contain between 50 and 100 international units of vitamin E, take an extra vitamin E supplement to bring your total intake up to 100 milligrams. D-alpha tocopherol is the most active vitamin E available. Be careful not to take more vitamins than you need—1,600 international units or more of vitamin E has been shown to depress immunity.

HIGH BLOOD PRESSURE (HYPERTENSION)

When a health professional takes your blood pressure, he or she is actually assessing the strength of the force exerted by the flow of blood against the arteries. Blood is pumped from the heart to the rest of the body via the arteries and returns to the heart through the veins. The connectors that join the arteries and the veins are the arterioles, which control blood pressure.

Blood pressure is expressed as the values of systolic pressure (the pressure exerted in the vessels when the heart contracts) over diastolic pressure (the pressure exerted when the heart relaxes)—for example, 120/80 mm Hg (milligrams of mercury). Blood pressure is considered to be high when it exceeds 140/90 in two or more readings. High blood pressure, also called hypertension, is dangerous because elevated blood pressure forces the heart to work harder. Also, it scars the arteries and decreases their elasticity, leading to an increased risk of heart attack or stroke.

Phytochemical-Rich Foods to Help Fight High Blood Pressure

While there are prescription medications prescribed to lower blood pressure, there are foods that will help prevent hypertension in the first place and help lower blood pressure if it is allowed to become elevated.

Garlic

Garlic may be helpful for keeping your blood pressure under control. When researchers combined the results of eight different studies, they concluded that people with high blood pressure who took garlic powder supplements every day for one month to one year lowered their systolic pressure by eight points and their diastolic pressure by an average of five points. Allicin is the phytochemical in garlic that is believed to be responsible. Food is the safest method of getting valuable phytochemicals, but if you are looking to purchase garlic supplements, pay attention to the number of pills needed to provide the same amount of allicin—5,000 micrograms—in one-third teaspoon of garlic powder.

When using fresh garlic, mincing is better than slicing. The more cuts you make, the more allicin you get. Although cooking may destroy some of the valuable compounds, light cooking may make the garlic less apt to irritate sensitive stomachs and mouths. One or two cloves daily of fresh, slightly cooked garlic may help in the battle against hypertension.

Celery

In one documented case, eating one-quarter pound of celery daily lowered the blood pressure of a man with mild hypertension from 158/96 mm Hg to a normal level of 118/82 mm Hg. Among herbalists, celery has a reputation for acting as a diuretic and has been used in East Asian folk medicine for centuries to treat high blood pressure.

Researchers were able to decrease the blood pressure of lab animals by 12 to 14 percent by injecting them with phthalide, a phytochemical present in celery. Phthalide, which is responsible for the distinctive flavor of celery, decreased the amount of catecholamines in the blood of the test animals. Catecholamines are the stress hormones in the blood that cause blood vessels to constrict, increasing blood pressure.

Dietary Recommendations

Data from a multicenter research study developed at Harvard University, which were reported at the annual meeting of the American Heart Association in 1996, showed that an easy-to-follow diet, high in plant foods, can be as beneficial as medicine for lowering blood pressure. Four hundred and fifty-nine people with high and moderately high blood pressure participated in the study. Within a matter of days, blood pressure was reduced by 11.4 over 5.5 points in those with high blood pressure and 3.5 over 2.1 in those with normal blood pressure. All participants had systolic pressure of less than 160 and diastolic pressure of 80 to 90. These results are as good as those achieved with the medications used to treat hypertension, and the diet is flexible and easy to follow—everyone who started the study was able to see it through to the finish. This eating plan is detailed below. However, don't stop taking your medications before consulting your health-care provider.

To accomplish the eating plan to lower high blood pressure, include ten standard servings of fruits and vegetables in your diet daily. If you're eating the "five-a-day" servings of fruits and vegetables that Americans have been urged to eat, double your portion sizes to reach ten servings per day. Eat seven to eight servings of grains and grain products daily.

Maintain the calories from fat at 27 percent or fewer of the total calories eaten. Space your fat grams out across your meals throughout the day. Maintain calories from saturated fat at 6 percent of calories eaten. Those who achieved success with the trial diet didn't exceed two 6-ounce servings of roasted or broiled skinless lean meats, fish, or poultry daily. Instead, have four to five servings a week of cooked beans, nuts, or seeds. In general, limit added fats to no more than two to three servings a day. That translates into no more than three teaspoons or pats of butter or oil daily. When using prepared salad dressing, one tablespoon of regular, or two tablespoons of low-fat, dressing can be substituted for one teaspoon of oil. Two teaspoons of mayonnaise can be substituted for one pat of oil or margarine. Have two to three servings of low-fat or nonfat dairy products daily.

Maintain a moderate salt intake. Intake of sodium should not exceed 3,000 milligrams daily, as even this much is more salt than experts previously recommended for a diet to lower high blood pressure. Limit foods with 480 milligrams of sodium or more per serving to one serving a day. Some people are salt-sensitive and some are not. For people who are salt-sensitive, a reduction of sodium will be followed by decreased blood pressure, if blood pressure was elevated. For some people, decreasing salt intake will make little difference. There is still no simple test you can take to determine salt sensitivity.

Limit sweets to five servings a week. You may include one tablespoon five times a week of maple syrup, sugar, jelly, or jam. Sweet snacks that fit the bill are fifteen jellybeans, three pieces of hard candy, or one-half cup of fruit gelatin.

Though there are a lot of components to this diet, the secret to its success may be in the increased intake of phytochemicals from the ten servings of fruits and vegetables daily.

In addition, avoid natural licorice. It contains glycyrrhizic acid, which increases the body's ability to retain water. Approximately 100 grams of natural licorice enhances sodium reabsorption, which increases blood pressure.

Suggested Lifestyle Changes

If you are overweight, lose weight. As little as ten pounds of weight lost can reduce blood pressure. There is an increase of blood pressure of 6.6 milliliters of mercury for every 10 percent of weight gain over ideal body weight.

Limit your alcohol intake. Those people following the diet to lower high blood pressure kept their intake at one to two drinks a week. A drink of alcohol is considered five ounces of wine, twelve ounces of beer, or one-and-one-half ounces of eighty-proof distilled spirits.

Sample Menu for a Blood-Pressure-Lowering Diet

Here's a sample of a day's menu for a person who needs to consume 2,000 calories to maintain his or her weight. Depending on your caloric needs, adjust the serving amounts proportionately.

Food	Amount	Servings
BREAKFAST		
Orange juice	6 ounces (60 calories)	1 fruit
Milk, skim or 1-percent low-fat	8 ounces (90 calories)	1 dairy
Cheerios with 1 tsp. sugar	1 cup (100 calories)	2 grains
Banana	1 medium (100 calories)	1 fruit
Whole-wheat bread	1 slice (80 calories)	1 grain
Margarine or butter	1 teaspoon (45 calories)	1 fat
LUNCH		
Sliced turkey	3 ounces (150 calories)	1 meat
Whole-wheat bread	2 slices (80 calories)	2 grains
Lettuce and tomato	2 slices each (25 calories)	1 vegetable
Carrot sticks	6 sticks (25 calories)	1 vegetable
Grapes	½ cup (60 calories)	1 fruit
Milk, skim or 1-percent low-fat	8 ounces (90 calories)	1 dairy

If you are sedentary, get thirty to forty-five minutes of aerobic exercise at least three times a week. Start with walking and ask your doctor if more vigorous exercise would be beneficial.

If you smoke, stop. Nicotine constricts the blood vessels, increasing blood pressure.

DINNER		
Vegetable juice	6 ounces (40 calories)	1 vegetable
Baked salmon fillet	3 ounces (40 calories)	1 fish
Brown or white rice pilaf	1 cup (160 calories)	2 grains
Broccoli, cooked with garlic and olive oil	½ cup (25 calories)	1 vegetable, ½ fat
Romaine lettuce salad with mixed raw veggies	1 cup (25 calories)	1 vegetable
Light salad dressing	1 tablespoon (25 calories)	½ fat
Strawberries	½ cup (60 calories)	1 fruit
SNACKS		
Cinnamon toast with 1 tsp. honey and 1 tsp. margarine	2 slices (160 calories)	2 grains, 1 fat
Raisins	¼ cup (108 calories)	1 fruit
Peanuts	⅓ cup (275 calories)	1 serving nuts
Diet soda	12 ounces	Free calories

If you need more or less calories to achieve your weight goals, adjust the above menu proportionately for your needs. If you prefer butter to margarine, use skim milk instead of one-percent milk and you will keep your saturated fat intake where it belongs.

Human Papilloma Virus (HPV)

Human papilloma virus (HPV) is a sexually transmitted infection. There are at least sixty different types of HPVs. Some HPVs cause cauliflower-shaped growths or warts that frequently appear in the genital region. A wide variety of benign and malignant growths may be associated with HPV, which also causes other genital infections that are not visible.

HPV also is responsible for recurrent papilloma growths in the upper respiratory tract that block the airway and impede breathing. Frequent surgical removal of these growths is often necessary to maintain an adequate opening in the airway to sustain life.

It is believed that HPV stays in the body for life like the herpes and hepatitis viruses. Although some people's experience with the growths caused by HPV have been limited to one outbreak, some people have recurring outbreaks. There is no permanent cure for HPV. The only known treatment for growths caused by HPV is surgery or chemical removal.

Phytochemical-Rich Foods to Fight the Human Papilloma Virus

The human papilloma virus is stimulated by estrogen. The indole-3-carbinol (I3C) content of cabbage and other cruciferous vegetables has demonstrated the ability to stop the growth of recurrent respiratory papilloma caused by HPV due to its capacity to alter estrogen metabolism. In one recently published study, 200 milligrams of pure indole-3-carbinol was effective in keeping 70 percent of fifty children with recurrent respiratory papillomas in remission. Indole-3-carbinol is available in supplement form. Four cups of uncooked cabbage or broccoli can provide approximately 100 milligrams of I3C. Studies are under way that will test the ability of indole-3-carbinol from cruciferous vegetables to impede the growth of genital warts. Daily ingestion of four to six ounces of cabbage juice extracted from eight to twelve ounces of cabbage has stopped the growth of recurrent respiratory papillomas in children.

MENOPAUSE

Menopause is not an illness but a natural condition that occurs in women around the beginning of the fifth decade of life when reproductive function slows down. It is marked by decreased amounts of the reproductive hormones estrogen and progesterone and also can be surgically induced by the removal of the ovaries.

The scarcity of estrogen at menopause is thought to be responsible for menopausal symptoms, including night sweats, hot flashes, vaginal dryness, and pain during intercourse. Even more troubling than the short-term discomforts are the disorders that reportedly occur as an effect of the decreased levels of estrogen—cardiovascular disorders and osteoporosis.

Although 80 to 90 percent of American women report some discomfort from symptoms of menopause, the unpleasant side effects of decreased estrogen production are not universally noted phenomena. Asian women who eat the traditional Asian diet report far fewer of the annoying symptoms of menopause than American women do. It is thought that their diet, which is low in fat and rich in vegetables and soybeans, offers them hormonelike phytochemicals, often referred to as phytoestrogens, which shield them from the troubling discomforts of menopause. Phytoestrogens are estrogenlike phytochemicals that are thought to act as a proxy for human estrogen by attaching to estrogen receptor molecules and providing a weak estrogenlike surrogate.

Phytochemical-Rich Foods That May Help Fight the Symptoms of Menopause

There exists a bounty of phytochemical-rich foods that appears to help women manage the symptoms of menopause. In addition to providing sustenance and phytoestrogens, they can provide women with the ability to be proactive in managing their own health.

Legumes

Legumes, particularly soybeans, are good sources of phytoestrogens. Research that evaluates the effect of soy foods on the symptoms of menopause is conflicting but also promising. A recent Italian study found that when menopausal women ate 40 grams of soy protein (equivalent to about six ounces of tofu) daily for twelve weeks, they reported 45 percent fewer hot flashes than before eating the soy. But other women given the same amount of milk protein for twelve weeks reported 30 percent fewer hot flashes, suggesting that hot flashes are subject to a strong placebo effect (an improvement in a subject's symptoms due to the patient's expectations of the therapy rather than a response to the therapy itself). Other studies have shown a decrease in quantity and duration of hot flashes with 45 to 90 milligrams of soy isoflavones, the amount found in two to three servings of soy foods. Foods made from soybeans can be helpful in controlling the symptoms of menopause due to their high content of the isoflavones genistein and daidzein, which act as phytoestrogens. About 45 milligrams of soy isoflavones may begin to offer relief from symptoms of menopause.

When it comes to the long-range consequences of decreased estrogen on women's health, the data on the value of soy foods are favorable. More than thirty years of research has shown that the inclusion of soy protein in the diet can lower serum cholesterol significantly. Intakes of 25 to 50 grams of soy protein daily can result in a 10-percent drop in heart-damaging low-density-lipoprotein cholesterol levels. Researchers claim that of all the potential benefits that soy phytoestrogens might offer, reducing osteoporosis risk holds the most promise. Isoflavones reduce bone breakdown and stimulate bone formation, whereas estrogen only inhibits bone breakdown. One animal study and three short-term studies on postmenopausal women show that soy isoflavones help to reduce bone loss.

You may find that the research on isoflavones found in legumes is dominated by references to soy foods. Soybeans are slightly higher in total isoflavone content than other beans, but I would be remiss if I did not point out that most legumes, including black beans, kidney beans, pinto beans, lentils, and lima beans all are rich sources of isoflavones and can promote a healthy menopause.

Flaxseeds

Flaxseeds contain lignans, which are rich sources of phytoestrogens. Although lignans also are found in whole grains, nuts, and other seeds, the richest known source of lignans is the flaxseed. Flaxseed has 750 to 800 times as much lignan as the nearest runner-up, the lentil. In one study, three groups of postmenopausal women supplemented their diets with 45 grams of soy flour, 25 grams of flaxseed, or 10 grams of red clover seed sprouts. Researchers then determined the maturity of their vaginal cells and found that the cells matured significantly after supplementation with soy flour and flaxseed but not after supplementation with the red clover seed sprouts. Many menopausal women experience painful intercourse due to thinning of the lining of the vagina. This research showed that the cell structure of the vaginal wall could be improved with flaxseed supplementation due to flaxseed's estrogenic quality.

Other Dietary Recommendations

If excessive menstrual bleeding is a problem, make sure to eat foods rich in vitamin C, because ascorbic acid and bioflavonoids help to promote collagen formation needed for healthy cell membranes. When eating whole citrus fruits, be sure to eat some of the white membrane to boost your intake of bioflavonoids, which are necessary for cell membrane integrity.

Use whole-grain products like whole-wheat bread, brown rice, and whole oats to boost the lignan content of your diet and reduce your risk of death from heart attack, as postmenopausal women lose some protection against cardiovascular disease when estrogen production ceases. Cardiovascular disease is the number-one killer of women.

Many menopausal women report that alcoholic beverages, even in small amounts, trigger hot flashes and night sweats. Coffee, particularly hot coffee, is reported by menopausal women to also trigger hot flashes.

Suggested Supplements

Some women find relief from hot flashes and night sweats by taking a vitamin E supplement. For this purpose, 800 international units may be helpful; however, more than 1,600 international units of vitamin E have been shown to depress immunity.

If your diet does not provide 1,200 milligrams of calcium, consider using calcium carbonate or calcium citrate supplements to make up the difference to help prevent osteoporosis. Sometimes, all it takes to make up the shortfall is a glass of calcium-fortified orange juice daily. Of course, you also should be sure to include at least a glass of skim or one-percent milk and other dairy products in your diet.

Some General Recommendations

Increase any behavior that you notice diminishes menopausal symptoms and avoid situations that create or stimulate menopausal symptoms. Most women who exercise report fewer hot flashes than women who do not exercise. Keep a bottle of water handy. Some women report that a long drink of water at the start of a hot flash can help reduce its intensity. Many women also report that consumption of alcohol, particularly of wine, stimulates hot flashes. Dress in layers so that when you feel a hot flash coming, you can remove some outer clothing. Wear natural fibers because they breathe and keep you cooler. Keep the thermostat turned down, because the warmer the room is, the more intense the hot flash is likely to be. Avoid or limit caffeine and hot drinks, as these too may stimulate hot flashes.

OSTEOPOROSIS

"Osteoporosis" literally translated means "porous bones." It is a disease in which bones become fragile and are more likely to break. Osteoporosis is painless until a bone breaks—typically in the hip, spine, or wrist. One in two women and one in eight men will break a bone due to osteoporosis.

Bone mass is always changing. We are constantly accumulating and utilizing bone mass. There is a constant state of flux between bone that is being created from calcium and collagen and bone that is being broken down or resorbed. Until about the age of thirty or thirty-five, the accumulation outweighs the utilization, putting us in a positive state of bone balance. After the age of thirty-five, we no longer increase bone mass, but we continue to draw on the balance. As part of the natural process of aging, bone breaks down faster than it can be built. In women, bone loss occurs faster than it can be built after menopause as a result of decreased estrogen levels. Estrogen protects against bone loss. Osteoporosis tends to occur ten years earlier in women than men because men typically have larger bones and more bone mass from which to draw.

Assessing Your Risk of Developing Osteoporosis

Since osteoporosis is silent and painless until a fracture occurs, it is important to know if you are at increased risk of developing the disease, so you can act aggressively to control any alterable risk factors. Early detection is important. If you are past the age of forty-five, ask your doctor about bone density testing. It is a painless, noninvasive procedure that will help you to better assess your risk for developing osteoporosis.

Risk Factors You Can't Change

1. *Gender.* Women tend to be more at risk than men are.

2. *Age.* The older you get, the higher your risk becomes.

3. *Body size.* Smaller-framed adults are considered at increased risk because they have less of a store of bone to draw from than larger-framed people.

4. *Ethnicity.* Caucasians are at increased risk of hip and vertebral fractures, and Asians are at increased risk of only vertebral fractures. African-Americans and Hispanics are at lower risk of fractures.

5. *Family history.* There may be a genetic predisposition to an increased risk of bone fracture.

(continued on page 160)

(continued from page 159)

Risk Factors You Can Change

1. *Sex hormones.* With a decrease in the amount of circulating sex hormones, there is an increased amount of bone loss and risk of fracture.

2. *Anorexia.* A history of anorexia influences bone mass and increases the risk of fractures.

3. *Nutrition history.* A low lifetime intake of calcium and vitamin D appears to influence the density of bone mass and increases the risk of fracture.

4. *Pharmaceuticals.* Certain medicines like glucocorticoids (cortisone) and certain anticonvulsants increase the risk of fracture.

5. *Inactive lifestyle.* Inactive lifestyle or extensive bed rest can decrease bone mass and increase the risk of fractures.

6. *Cigarette smoking.* Cigarette smoking destroys vitamin C, which is needed for the formation of collagen, an essential component of bones.

7. *Alcohol.* Extensive use of alcohol increases the risk of decreased bone mass and bone fracture.

8. *History of periodontal disease.* There is a strong association between the presence of periodontal disease and the risk of osteoporosis. The loss of mineral content in the teeth makes them and the surrounding area more susceptible to periodontal disease.

Phytochemical-Rich Foods That Can Help You Fight Osteoporosis

Lately, women have been advised to take calcium supplements to increase their bone strength. This is, of course, sound advice; however, there are dietary changes that women can and should make that also will promote bone health.

Legumes

Legumes, particularly soybeans, are rich in genistein, the isoflavone that is most active in its ability to bind to estrogen receptors. Research from a six-month clinical trial compared bone density in three groups of postmenopausal women. Those who received 40 grams of soy protein containing 80 milligrams of soy isoflavones a day experienced an increase in bone mineral density. Studies that examine bone density over at least a two-year period are needed to confirm the apparent findings. Some studies suggest that genistein inhibits bone breakdown, and others show that isoflavones stimulate bone formation. Animal studies show that soymilk accelerates intestinal calcium absorption. If you are depending on tofu as a source of calcium, check the label to ensure that calcium is added. It is often used to set the tofu into a firm consistency. Adding two to three ounces of legumes a day to your diet is a good start to promoting bone health.

Flaxseeds

Another edible source of phytoestrogen is flaxseed. Flaxseed contains lignans, which can help the body produce its own estrogenlike substance that may help to decrease the bone loss that occurs after menopause when estrogen levels decrease. Twenty-five grams a day have been used to reverse other negative side effects of menopause.

Calcium-Rich Vegetables

Broccoli, kale, and collard greens all are fair sources of calcium in addition to being rich in many anticancer compounds. It previously was believed that chemicals in vegetables called oxalates and phytates reduced the availability of calcium from plants in the body. More recent studies, however, have shown that the percentage of calcium from kale and broccoli absorbed by the body is greater than the percentage of calcium absorbed from dairy foods.

Other Dietary Recommendations

It is recommended that you get between 1,000 and 1,500 milligrams of calcium daily and between 400 and 600 international units (IU) of vitamin D. To reach the upper limits of that recommendation, shoot for three to four servings of dairy products or calcium-rich foods daily. Milk, unlike other dairy products, is fortified with vitamin D. Four glasses of milk a day should provide the recommended 400 international units of vitamin D and approximately 1,200 milligrams of calcium. Incidental food intake will account for about 200 milligrams of calcium. If your calcium intake is on the low side, to minimize calcium loss, try to reduce your intake of such foods as coffee, sodium, and animal protein, which slightly increase calcium excretion.

Suggested Lifestyle Changes

Lifestyle factors play as important a role as diet does in preventing osteoporosis. Exercise and exposure to sunlight are very important factors in maintaining bone mass. The National Academy of Sciences recommends 400 international units (IU) of vitamin D for people ages fifty-one to seventy and 600 international units (IU) for people ages seventy-one or older for maximum bone health. Most foods have little or no vitamin D. It is created in the skin when it is exposed to ultraviolet light. Sunscreen with sun protection factor (SPF) prevents your body from producing active vitamin D.

To help maintain bone health, engage in weight-bearing exercise regularly. Strive for thirty minutes a day. Walking, dancing, and aerobics all are good choices. The important thing is that you enjoy whatever you choose. If you do not enjoy an activity, statistics show that you will not stay with it. Try meeting a friend for a walk regularly. Rather than planning a lunch date, plan a walk date. It meets two important needs: the need for socialization and the need for exercise. A stroll in the summer also will help you to get the vitamin D you need to help build bone.

Suggested Supplements

Even if you take a multivitamin/mineral supplement, you may find that you are not getting all the calcium you need. Calcium molecules are large, and manufacturers can't pack much of it into a multivitamin/mineral pill. If you feel you are not meeting your needs with food, try to make up the difference between what you need and what you get from foods with a supplement. Supplements come in many forms. Calcium-fortified orange juice can act as a food supplement. An eight-ounce glass of fortified juice will provide as much calcium as an eight-ounce glass of milk. Calcium carbonate and calcium citrate malate are both well-absorbed supplements, available in tablet form. Look for a calcium supplement that includes vitamin D, which is also needed to build bones. The National Academy of Sciences recommends 400 international units (IU) of vitamin D for people ages fifty-one to seventy and 600 international units (IU) for people ages seventy-one or older for maximum bone health. According to the National Academy of Sciences, the tolerable upper limit for calcium supplements is 2,500 milligrams daily. Vitamin D intake should not exceed 2,000 international units for adults.

PREMENSTRUAL SYNDROME

Premenstrual syndrome (PMS) is a predictable pattern of physical and emotional changes that occurs monthly prior to menstruation in 40 to 60 percent of women during the childbearing years. The most frequently reported physical symptoms include bloating, fluid retention, weight gain, and breast soreness. Emotional changes include irritability, anxiety, mood swings, and depression.

It is believed that PMS is caused by the changes in hormone levels that occur during a woman's menstrual cycle. Women who report symptoms of PMS are thought to have high levels of blood estrogen as compared with progesterone, the other female hormone largely present during the childbearing years. PMS could possibly be referred to as estrogen intoxication.

Since the early 1980s when PMS was named, many women have

reported relief from their symptoms by instituting a variety of nutritional and lifestyle changes.

Phytochemical-Rich Foods That Help Fight PMS

Legumes, such as soy foods, flaxseeds, and certain whole grains, which are rich in lignans, could be very useful in reducing the levels of potent circulating estrogen in women with an abundant estrogen supply. The isoflavones and lignans in beans and whole grains will compete with a woman's own estrogen for attachment to estrogen receptors. Plant estrogen compounds have the powerful ability to attach to estrogen receptors but are milder acting than human estrogen. Competition for attachment to estrogen receptors should displace self-made estrogen and should result in a weaker, less toxic pool of estrogen circulating in the female body. In studies on premenopausal women, phytoestrogen-rich diets significantly prolonged the postmenstruation phase of the menstrual cycle from fifteen to seventeen-and-a-half days, decreasing estrogen exposure.

Women of childbearing age might be cautioned not to overuse phytoestrogens and plant lignans because it is possible that temporary infertility can be caused by an overuse of plant estrogens. For example, animals grazing in pastures on crops that were later found to have estrogenic activity have displayed decreased rates of pregnancy. However, eating phytoestrogens in foods should cause no problem, as large parts of the world's population depend heavily on phytoestrogen-rich foods, namely the soybean, for sustenance, without reports of abnormally high rates of infertility. Good advice is to follow the model of the typical Asian diet. On average, Asians consume 1.5 to 2 milligrams of soy isoflavones per kilogram of body weight daily. To determine how much is best for you, divide your weight in pounds by 2.2 and then multiply that figure by 1.75.

Other Dietary Recommendations

There is a significant amount of anecdotal information that supports the adoption of dietary changes to help alleviate the symptoms of premenstrual syndrome. If you are overweight, striving to achieve and maintain an ideal body weight can be helpful because the loss of body fat would help reduce the amount of estrogen being stored by the fat cells of the body.

Emphasis should be placed on a diet high in whole grains, fruits, and vegetables; moderate in protein; and relatively low in simple carbohydrates that come from sugar and refined flour products.

Monitor your intake of fat from animal sources like meat and cheese. A reduction in calories coming from animal fat would help to reduce the amount of prostaglandin 2 made by the body. Prostaglandins are hormonelike substances made and used by body tissue. High levels of prostaglandin 2 have been linked to menstrual cramps and an imbalance of the estrogen/progesterone levels favoring increased estrogen. Vegetarians who eat high-fiber diets excrete more estrogen in their feces and have 50-percent less circulating conjugated blood estrogen (a type of metabolized estrogen) than do women who eat meat.

A reduction in caffeine-containing products, including coffee, tea, cola, and chocolate, could help to reduce breast soreness, as caffeine is believed to be an exacerbating culprit in benign fibrocystic breast disease.

Suggested Lifestyle Changes

Engage in aerobic exercise at least three times a week for a minimum of twenty to thirty minutes. Research confirms that exercise increases endorphins in the blood, nature's own opiates that impart a feeling of well-being and help to dispel depression and anxiety.

If exercise alone does not relieve anxiety, consider engaging in stress-reduction techniques like yoga or meditation. To experience the effects of yoga in your own living room, consider renting the videotape *Yoga Moves* by Allen Finger. It will give you a good idea of what yoga is about. To learn meditation techniques, review the book *The Relaxation Response* by Dr. Herbert Benson.

Suggested Supplements

A good multivitamin and mineral with about 50 milligrams of the B-complex vitamins will ensure that you are getting an adequate supply of the B vitamins. If it does not provide 100 international units (IU) of vitamin E, use an additional supplement to reach that total. In a recent multicenter study, 1,200 milligrams of calcium carbonate eliminated the majority of premenstrual syndrome symptoms in 50 percent of 500 women. Many women found gamma-linoleic acid (GLA) in the form of borage oil, black currant oil, or evening primrose oil to be effective in helping to reduce symptoms of PMS. Generally, 500 milligrams is prescribed three to four times a day as an additional source of essential fatty acid. Nuts and seeds also could provide additional essential fatty acids.

General Recommendations

One way to determine if your health problems are caused by premenstrual syndrome is to keep a calendar or journal recording your moods, feelings, and general health. If a monthly pattern of "dis-ease" emerges that coincides with your menstrual cycle, you will have discovered valuable information that can help you put yourself on the road back to feeling well.

The concept of making dietary changes to alter the disease process is not new. For centuries, people have been using diet to fortify their health. What is new is the discovery of the way in which specific substances within plant foods assist the body in fending off disease. We can take this information and use it wisely by incorporating it into our health-care practice. Using phytochemicals to fight disease is cost-efficient and self-empowering. The challenge we are now faced with is finding as many opportunities as possible to incorporate phytochemical-rich foods into our lives.

Part III

Phytochemical-Rich Recipes

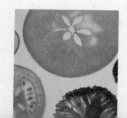

To make your diet more phytochemically rich, you don't really need a file of recipes. Fruits, vegetables, and many grains and legumes are among the easiest of foods to eat and prepare. Something as simple as tofu, carrot sticks, and broccoli florets would easily serve as a quick and easy phytochemical-rich meal. But you also can sauté the tofu, broccoli, and carrot sticks in some olive oil with a few scallions and soy sauce thickened with kuzu, and serve it over brown rice. Now *that's* a meal! These recipes will add a little variety to your meals and make them even more pleasurable. I hope you enjoy them. Each one is rich in phytochemicals and, just as important, delicious. *Bon appétit.*

Tasty Breakfast Treats

You've probably heard this one before: Breakfast is the most important meal of the day. That's because it's true. You probably can't be told often enough until you make a strict habit of eating breakfast every day. It does not have to be a traditional sit-down breakfast to be sufficient. Sometimes I make a bowl of Appley Oatmeal for One, put it in a container, and eat it when I get to work. What's important is that you get some protein, some carbohydrates, and maybe a little fat into your stomach before you try to take on the world each day. Go ahead. You'll feel better and be less apt to overeat at your other meals if you eat a good breakfast—and the breakfasts you'll find in this section are not only nutritious, they're tasty, too.

Cranberry Orange Muffins

I usually feel inclined to whip up a batch of muffins around Thanks-giving when cranberries are plentiful and likely to be in the house. They are especially good served warm from the oven. These little gems contain lignans along with some limonene since they combine flaxseed with the rind of the citrus fruit.

YIELD: 14 MUFFINS

1¾ cups unbleached flour

3 tablespoons ground flaxseed (a small coffee grinder works well for grinding the seeds)

1½ teaspoons baking powder

½ teaspoon baking soda

½ teaspoon salt

Juice and grated rind of one orange

2 tablespoons melted butter

About 2 to 3 tablespoons boiling water

1 medium egg

¼ cup honey

¾ cup maple syrup

1 cup coarsely chopped cranberries

1½ cups chopped pecans, toasted

1. Preheat the oven to 400°F. If you are not using paper muffin cups, grease the muffin tin.

2. Sift together the flour, flaxseed, baking powder, baking soda, and salt in a large bowl. Set aside.

3. Place the orange juice and grated rind in a heatproof measuring cup. Add the melted butter and enough boiling water to make ¾ cup of liquid.

4. In a small bowl, beat the egg with a fork. Add the hot liquid to the egg, beating continuously to mix well. Add the honey and maple syrup.

5. Add the liquid mixture to the dry ingredients and mix them together. Mix in the cranberries and the pecans, if desired.

6. Fill each muffin tin ⅔ full and bake for 20 to 25 minutes, until golden. They should spring back when you gently poke them.

Nutritional information per muffin:

Calories: 215 (10 percent from fat)   **Carbohydrates:** 30 grams
Cholesterol: 19 milligrams   **Fat:** 2.8 grams   **Fiber:** 1.5 grams
Protein: 2.8 grams   **Sodium:** 150 milligrams

Lemon Poppy Seed Spa Muffins

These are delicious lower-fat versions of the lemon poppy seed muffins found in the bakery. Try them. You won't feel the least bit deprived.

YIELD: 12 MUFFINS

1¼ cups unbleached flour	½ cup nonfat plain yogurt
¾ cup whole-wheat flour	¼ cup honey
2 tablespoons poppy seeds	2 tablespoons maple syrup
2 teaspoons baking powder	¼ cup fresh lemon juice
1 teaspoon baking soda	3 tablespoons skim milk
½ teaspoon salt	1 tablespoon melted butter
1 egg	2 teaspoons grated lemon rind

1. Preheat the oven to 400°F. If you are not using paper muffin cups, grease the muffin tin.

2. Combine the dry ingredients in a large bowl.

3. In a separate bowl, blend the wet ingredients.

4. Stir the wet ingredients into the dry until just moistened. The batter will be thick.

5. Pour the batter into muffin tins. Bake for 18 to 20 minutes, until browned.

Nutritional information per muffin:

Calories: 138 (14.8 percent from fat)   **Carbohydrates:** 26 grams
Cholesterol: 20 milligrams   **Fat:** 2.27 grams   **Fiber:** 1 gram
Proteins: 3.5 grams   **Sodium:** 282 grams

Peaches and Cream Couscous

This dish makes a delightful summer breakfast. Double the recipe for a breakfast for two.

YIELD: 1 SERVING

1 cup water

½ cup couscous

1 sliced ripe peach

1 teaspoon honey

A pinch of nutmeg

About 3 tablespoons evaporated skim or soy milk

1. In a small pot, bring the water to a boil, add couscous, peach slices, and honey, and stir. Cook at low heat for about 2 minutes. Cover. Let sit until the water is absorbed (about 5 to 10 minutes).

2. Add the milk. Dust with nutmeg before serving.

Nutritional information per serving:

Calories: 153 (6 percent from fat)   **Carbohydrates:** 30 grams
Cholesterol: 0 milligrams   **Fat:** 1 gram   **Fiber:** 1 gram
Protein: 3 grams   **Sodium:** 15 grams

Appley Oatmeal for One

I love this oatmeal. You can increase the phytochemical content by stirring in a tablespoon of ground flaxseed after it is cooked.

YIELD: 1 SERVING

¾ cup water

⅓ cup whole oats

½ medium Macintosh apple, unpeeled, diced

⅛ teaspoon cinnamon

2 teaspoons maple syrup

About 3 tablespoons soymilk

1. Heat the water in a small pot. Add the oats and diced apple. Cook uncovered over low heat for 3 minutes.

2. Add the cinnamon and maple syrup. Let it sit covered for about 5 minutes.

3. Add the soymilk and enjoy.

Variation: Eliminate the maple syrup and add a chopped date or two. The date will melt into the oatmeal, lending sufficient sweetness to the dish.

Nutritional information per muffin:

Calories: 184 (about 15 percent from fat)   **Cholesterol:** 0 milligrams
Carbohydrates: 36 grams   **Fat:** 3 grams   **Fiber:** 5 grams
Protein: 5.6 grams   **Sodium:** 8 milligrams

Flaxen Oatmeal Muffins

These muffins are moist and slightly sweet. They are especially good when served warm from the oven, but just as good one day old.

YIELD: 12 MUFFINS

1 cup yogurt	¼ cup honey
1 cup rolled oats	1 cup unbleached flour
1 medium egg	2 tablespoons ground flaxseed
2 tablespoons melted butter	½ teaspoon baking soda
2 tablespoons canola oil	1 teaspoon baking powder
2 tablespoons maple syrup	½ teaspoon salt

1. Preheat the oven to 400°F. If you are not using paper muffin cups, grease the muffin tin.

2. Mix together the yogurt and oats in a small bowl. Let this mixture sit for one hour.

3. In a large separate bowl, beat the egg. Then mix in the butter, oil, syrup, and honey.

4. In another small bowl, sift together the flours, baking powder, and salt.

5. Alternately add the flour mixture and the oat mixture to the egg mixture until they are entirely mixed. Pour mixture into muffin tins and bake for 20 to 25 minutes until golden brown.

Nutritional information per muffin:

Calories: 143 (29 percent from fat)   **Cholesterol:** 36 milligrams
Carbohydrates: 27 grams   **Fat:** 5.3 grams   **Fiber:** 1.5 grams
Protein: 6 grams   **Sodium:** 200 milligrams

Phytochemically Super Soups

 Soups are a great way to add variety to the way you serve vegetables. A large bowl of vegetable soup can take the place of a vegetable in a busy dinner when a burger or a sandwich is the main course.

Miso Soup 101

I developed a fondness for miso soup from eating at Japanese restaurants. It is easy enough to make, but not as simple as I initially thought. The first time I decided to try making it at home, I mixed a package of miso with a cup of boiling water. It didn't quite turn out like the miso soup I was served at the restaurant. I then set out to learn how to make it taste delicious at home. Here are the fruits of my labor.

YIELD: 4 SERVINGS

4 cups water

1 4-inch piece of Kombu (seaweed)* or 2 sheets of Nori (seaweed)*

1 shiitake mushroom, thinly sliced

1 tablespoon bonito flakes*

⅓ pound firm tofu, cubed

3 tablespoons miso

3 tablespoons thinly sliced scallion

*The seaweed and bonito flakes are available in the macrobiotic section of the health-food store.

1. In a medium saucepan, combine the water, seaweed, and mushrooms. Bring to a boil and let it boil for 4 minutes. Remove from heat. Add the bonito flakes, and let the mixture sit for 4 minutes.

2. Strain the soup. Add the cubed tofu, and simmer over low heat for 5 minutes.

3. Remove from heat, and thoroughly stir in the miso.

4. Pour soup into four bowls, and garnish with scallions. Serve hot.

Nutrition information per serving:

Calories: 64   Carbohydrates: less than two grams   Cholesterol: 0 milligrams
Fat: 3 grams   Fiber: less than 1 gram   Protein: 5 grams
Sodium: 470 milligrams

Smoker's Soup

I call this recipe "Smoker's Soup" because it offers a generous serving of watercress—the vegetable known for its PEITC content, which appears to inactivate the most potent toxin in nicotine.

YIELD: 8 SERVINGS

6–7 cups water

1 cup cooked white beans

1–2 onions, peeled and cut into 1-inch chunks

1–2 medium potatoes, peeled and cut into 1-inch chunks

2 carrots cut in chunks

1 chopped leek (with tough outer leaves discarded)

½ pound watercress washed and chopped

1 teaspoon dried basil

2 cloves minced garlic

3 tablespoons olive oil

Salt and pepper to taste

1. In a large pot, combine the water, beans, onions, potatoes, carrots, leek, watercress, and basil and cook for 20 minutes until the vegetables are tender.

2. Let the soup cool, and purée it in a blender or food processor or put it through a food mill. Return soup mixture to pot.

3. In a small frying pan, sauté the garlic in the olive oil for 1 to 2 minutes. Add to the puréed soup.

4. Season with salt and pepper to taste. For extra zip add hot sauce or umeboshi vinegar.

Nutritional information per serving:

Calories: 125 (36 percent from fat)   **Carbohydrates:** 13 grams
Cholesterol: 50 milligrams   **Fat:** 5 grams   **Fiber:** 3 grams   **Protein:** 3 grams
Sodium: 149 milligrams

Split Pea Soup Made Easy

This recipe is simple, delicious, inexpensive, and wholesome, and the ingredients are easy to find. By adding extra vegetables to this already healthy convenience food, you can make it more phytochemically dense than ever.

YIELD: 6 SERVINGS

1 tablespoon canola oil

2 carrots, peeled and diced

3 celery stalks (tops included), diced

1 large onion, diced

1 small parsnip, peeled and diced

1 6-ounce package split pea soup mix (usually found in the kosher aisle of the supermarket)

6 cups water

1. In a large, heavy soup pot, heat the oil over low heat. Add the vegetables. Stir to coat with the oil. Sauté for 5 minutes or until the onions are translucent. Cover the pot to sweat the vegetables.

2. Set aside the spice packet found in the soup package. Add the remaining ingredients of the soup mix to the pot. Cook for about 5 minutes over low heat.

3. Add the water to the pot. Cook for about 1 hour and 15 minutes. Add the contents of the spice packet. Cook for another 15 minutes. Remove from heat, and let the soup cool.

4. Purée the soup in a food processor in small batches at a time. Return soup to pot and reheat before serving.

Nutritional information per serving:

Calories: 155 (11.6 percent from fat)   **Carbohydrates:** 25 grams   **Fat:** 2 grams
Fiber: 5 grams   **Protein:** 8 grams   **Sodium:** 581 milligrams

Savory Side Dishes

 A main course is nothing without a side dish to complement it. These side dishes will spice up any meal. Some of them also make great appetizers, or even a delicious lunch or light dinner.

Sandwich Bread

This bread is moist and dense with just a touch of sweetness. It slices and freezes well. Preparing this bread is relatively mess-free and easy, as it requires no kneading and needs to rise only once.

YIELD: 3 LOAVES

2 cups water	3 cups whole-wheat flour
2 cups skim milk	2 teaspoons salt
½ cup molasses	2 eggs
¼ cup honey	¾ cup flax meal (ground flaxseed)
3 tablespoons dry yeast	4¾ cups unbleached white flour

1. Combine water, milk, molasses, and honey in a saucepan and heat at low heat. Add the yeast and mix well until yeast is dissolved.

2. In a large bowl, combine the whole-wheat flour and salt and add the yeast mixture. Add eggs and beat until smooth.

3. In a separate bowl, mix flax meal and white flour together. Then begin adding this flour mixture to the rest of the ingredients, stirring well to make a soft dough. This dough does not have to be kneaded.

4. Cover the bowl and let the dough rise in a warm place (about 85°F) until doubled (about 1½ hours).

5. Punch down the dough and divide it between three greased loaf pans. Do not let the bread rise again. Bake in a preheated 375°F oven for 35 to 40 minutes, until the loaves are nicely browned.

Nutritional information per serving:

Calories: 93 (9 percent from fat) **Carbohydrates:** 18 grams **Cholesterol:** 8 grams
Fat: less than 1 gram **Fiber:** 1.5 grams **Protein:** 3 grams
Sodium: 100 milligrams

Vegetarian Chopped Liver

This recipe is based on a traditional Jewish dairy recipe. I like this spread because it can be used as a tasty meatless sandwich filling or served with crackers as an appetizer.

YIELD: 2 CUPS (ABOUT 6 SERVINGS)

1 tablespoon canola oil

1 large onion, cut in half lengthwise and then thinly sliced into half-moon slices

½ teaspoon salt

1 9-ounce package of frozen string beans

½ cup walnuts, ground

3 hard-boiled eggs*

*Fat content of this recipe can be reduced by using 3 egg whites and only 1 or 2 yolks.

1. Heat the oil in a medium frying pan over low heat. Add the onions and stir to coat with oil. Sauté the onions for 3 minutes.

2. Cover the pan and continue cooking the onions about 10 minutes or until golden and very tender. Add the salt.

3. Cook the beans as directed on package until tender.

4. With the metal blade of a food processor, process all ingredients together until smooth.

5. Chill in refrigerator for 2 hours before serving.

6. Add pepper to taste.

Nutritional information per serving:

Calories: 135 **Carbohydrates:** 7 grams **Cholesterol:** 106 milligrams
Fat: 10 grams **Fiber:** 2.4 grams **Protein:** 4.5 grams
Sodium: 209 milligrams

Twice-Baked Potatoes with Tofu

These potatoes are a good way to introduce tofu to your family if they are a bit reluctant to try it.

YIELD: 4 SERVINGS

4 Yukon Gold potatoes, approximately 2 inches around

2-inch slice tofu, mashed

2 tablespoons milk

1 tablespoon butter or margarine

Salt and pepper to taste

1. Bake potatoes in 400°F for about 1 hour, until tender. Cut them in half and scoop out the contents, being careful not to damage the potato jackets.

2. Mash the potato innards with a fork and add the mashed tofu, milk, butter, and salt and pepper. Fill the potato jackets with the mixture. Bake on a cookie sheet for 10 to 15 minutes in a 350°F oven.

Note: If you'd like, the potatoes can be made ahead of time and stored in the refrigerator before baking the second time. Remove them from the refrigerator 20 minutes before cooking, and bake them 15 minutes before serving. For a variation, sprinkle the top with Parmesan cheese before baking.

Nutritional information per serving:

Calories: 190 (19 percent from fat)   **Carbohydrates:** 40 grams
Cholesterol: 8.2 milligrams   **Fat:** 4 grams   **Fiber:** 2.3 grams
Protein: 5 grams   **Sodium:** 54 grams

Mary's Tofu and Miso Hors d'oeuvres

My friend Mary is renowned for her parties, particularly the food. When she attends a "bring-a-dish" party, this dish is the one most requested by the host or hostess.

YIELD: 8 SERVINGS

1 tablespoon sesame seeds, toasted

¼ teaspoon salt

1½ tablespoons white miso*

8 ounces firm tofu

3 scallions, minced

*Can be found in health-food stores.

1. With a mortar and pestle or an electric coffee grinder, grind the sesame seeds with the salt. Add the miso and set aside.

2. Drop the tofu in boiling water for about 5 minutes. This gives the tofu a chewier texture.

3. Remove the tofu from the water and mash in a bowl. Add the sesame seed mixture and mix well. Sprinkle scallions on top.

This faux pâté is best served surrounded with crackers for scooping or spreading.

Nutritional information per 2-tablespoon serving:

Calories: 44 (32 percent from fat) **Carbohydrates:** 1 gram
Cholesterol: 0 milligrams **Fat:** 1.6 grams **Fiber:** less than 1 gram
Protein: 4 grams **Sodium:** 197 milligrams

Sweet Potato Casserole

This recipe was updated from an old southern favorite. Sweet potatoes are good any time of the year, but this method of preparation makes them a really special treat—truly appropriate for Thanksgiving dinner. If you want to decrease the fat content, halve or eliminate the nut topping.

YIELD: 12 SERVINGS

3 large sweet potatoes	1 teaspoon vanilla extract
2 eggs, slightly beaten	½ teaspoon salt
½ cup maple syrup	1 cup chopped pecans
½ stick butter	
⅓ cup soymilk or evaporated skim milk	

1. Bake the potatoes in a 400°F oven until soft, about 45 minutes. When they are cool enough to handle, remove and discard the skins. Mash the potatoes with a fork or potato masher.

2. Mix in the remaining ingredients except the pecans. Spread into a greased 1-quart casserole dish, top with pecans, and cover. Bake for 30 minutes. Uncover and bake an additional 5 minutes.

Nutritional information per serving:

Calories: 173 (60 percent from fat)   **Carbohydrates:** 15 grams
Cholesterol: 45 milligrams   **Fat:** 12 grams   **Fiber:** 3 grams
Protein: 2 grams   **Sodium:** 144 milligrams

Spicy Roasted Soybeans

These tasty treats make a good alternative to popcorn or chips. They also can be used in salads instead of croutons.

YIELD: 2 CUPS

2 cups soybeans that have been soaked in 3 cups of water for at least 8 hours

1 tablespoon canola oil

Salt to taste

Garlic powder to taste

Chili powder to taste

1. Lightly oil a cookie sheet with canola oil.

2. Drain beans and place on cookie sheet. Brush the beans with the remainder of oil. Sprinkle with salt, garlic, and chili powder.

3. Bake in a preheated 300°F oven for 30 minutes. Shake the pan at 15-minute intervals to prevent the soybeans from sticking. Soybeans should be lightly browned when done.

Nutritional information per 2-tablespoon serving:

Calories: 64 (70 percent from fat)   **Carbohydrates:** 4 grams
Cholesterol: 0 milligrams   **Fat:** 5 grams   **Fiber:** 1.2 grams
Protein: 4 grams   **Sodium:** 125 milligrams

Prosnut Butter™

USDA Botanist Dr. James Duke coined the phrase "prosnut butter" to name any combination of foods rich in beta-sitosterol (typically nut butters). To make a delicious "prosnut butter" concoction, add a handful or two of pumpkinseeds, Brazil nuts, or sunflower seeds to a small jar of prepared peanut butter. Spread it on an apple or whole-grain bread to create a tasty lunch or snack food.

Delicious Phytochemical-Rich Beverages

 Sometimes it is convenient to drink your phytochemicals, especially when you're on the run. Phytochemical-rich drinks also can add an extra phytochemical "punch" to your meals. Try one of these delicious drinks tonight.

Alcohol-Free Hot Toddy

This phytochemical cocktail can offer relief during cold and flu season. The ginger and cayenne pepper act to fight congestion, and the lemon gives it a boost of bioflavonoids and vitamin C.

YIELD: 1 SERVING

½ lemon

1½ cups water

1 tablespoon maple syrup

½ teaspoon grated ginger

Pinch cayenne pepper

1. Squeeze the juice from the lemon half into a small container. Set aside.

2. Pour the water in a small saucepan. Finely slice the lemon rind into slivers and add to the water. Simmer 10 minutes.

3. Strain the liquid into a cup or a mug. Add maple syrup and grated ginger along with the reserved lemon juice and the cayenne pepper.

Nutritional information per serving:

Calories: 52   **Carbohydrates:** 13 grams   **Cholesterol:** 0 grams   **Fat:** 0 grams
Fiber: 0 grams   **Protein:** 0 grams   **Sodium:** 2 grams

Kuzu Drink

This drink might be helpful for someone trying to kick an alcohol craving, due to its high content of isoflavones, particularly daidzein.

YIELD: 1 SERVING

1 tablespoon kuzu

1 cup water

1 tablespoon tamari (natural soy sauce)*

*Tamari can be purchased from an Asian foods store or health-food store.

1. Dissolve kuzu in 3 tablespoons of the water. Once the kuzu is dissolved, pour in the remaining water.

2. Heat over low heat, and stir until thickened.

3. Add tamari, and drink warm.

Nutritional information per serving:

Calories: 40   **Carbohydrates:** 8.1 grams   **Fat:** less than 1 gram
Fiber: less than 1 gram   **Protein:** 2 grams   **Sodium:** 1,005 milligrams

Cabbage Juice Cocktail

This recipe was borrowed from Cherie Calbom's *Juicing for Life*. This might be a good drink for those people struggling with human papilloma virus, as the cabbage is a good source of indole-3-carbinol.

YIELD: 1 SERVING

¼ head of cabbage

2 tomatoes

Push the cabbage and tomatoes through the hopper of a juicer and juice thoroughly.

Nutritional information per serving:

Calories: 86 (15 percent from fat)   **Carbohydrates:** 18 grams
Cholesterol: 0 milligrams   **Fat:** 1.5 grams   **Fiber:** less than 3 grams
Protein: 4 grams   **Sodium:** 57 grams

Phytochemical-Rich Main Courses to Please the Whole Family

 Most people responsible for preparing dinner for the family experience a moment of alarm during the day when they think, "Omigosh! What am I going to make for dinner tonight?" Usually, they are thinking it must be quick, healthy, and affordable, the ingredients must be easily accessible, and most of all—everyone should be able to enjoy it. These recipes were assembled with all of those factors in mind.

Mini Vegetable Lasagna

This recipe is another great way of introducing tofu to your children. It can be assembled ahead of time and stored in the refrigerator for a day or two before you are ready to bake and eat it.

YIELD: 3 TO 4 SERVINGS

Sauce
(2–3 cups jarred sauce can be substituted for recipe):

2 tablespoons olive oil

1 large onion

2 cloves garlic

1 28-ounce can crushed tomatoes

1 tablespoon tomato paste

1 cup water

1 teaspoon dried basil

1 teaspoon oregano

½ teaspoon salt

Filling:

¾ pound firm tofu, drained, patted dry, and mashed

4 ounces shredded part-skim milk mozzarella

½ teaspoon salt

Fresh ground pepper to taste

2 eggs

5 ounces frozen chopped spinach, thawed with the water squeezed out.

¼ cup Parmesan cheese

½ pound cooked lasagna noodles

To make the sauce:

1. Heat the oil in a heavy large pot over low heat. Add onion and garlic. Stir to coat. Cover pot to sweat vegetables. Cook 1 or 2 minutes.

2. Add can of crushed tomatoes. Cover and cook 20 minutes over low heat.

3. Add tomato paste, water, and spices. Cook 2 more hours with lid askew, stirring occasionally and adding extra water if necessary. Sauce can be made a day or two in advance and frozen if desired.

To make the filling:

1. In a large bowl, mix all of the filling ingredients except the noodles with a fork.

2. To assemble, coat the bottom of a 9-inch square brownie pan with about ½ cup sauce. Lay the noodles so that they are adjacent, but not touching. Spread filling mixture evenly. Cover with another ½ cup of sauce. Repeat process. Make sure you end up with lasagna noodles on top, covered with sauce. A little extra Parmesan or mozzarella cheese can be used on top if desired.

3. Cover with foil and bake 30 minutes in a 350°F oven. Uncover and bake 10 more minutes. Let it sit for 10 minutes covered before eating.

Nutritional information per serving:

Calories: 305 (30 percent from fat) **Carbohydrates:** 34 grams
Cholesterol: 122 milligrams **Fat:** 11 grams (saturated: 4 grams)
Fiber: 4.5 grams **Protein:** 20 grams **Sodium:** 465 milligrams

Black Bean Burrito or Taco Dinner

This dinner takes about 40 minutes to prepare. It gives the diners the choice to make up their own plate, choosing from a variety of foods. What I like best about this meal is that the meat-eater and the vegetarian can break bread together and not even view the gulf that exists between them. It consists of three hot choices: black beans, chopped turkey, and Spanish rice. In addition, the table is set with a variety of cold fixings.

YIELD: 5 SERVINGS

Beans:

½ pound dry black beans, or 2 cups canned black beans (reserve the liquid)

2 tablespoons olive oil

1 large onion, chopped

1 4-ounce jar pimentos

2 tablespoons wine

⅛ teaspoon oregano

½ teaspoon sugar

¼ teaspoon salt (if using canned beans, do not add salt)

1 small seeded chipotle pepper (smoked jalapeño), diced (optional)

Rice:

1 tablespoon olive oil

1 minced garlic clove

¾ cup chopped onion

1 teaspoon salt

1 teaspoon chili powder

1 cup brown rice

2 cups water

Ground turkey:

½ pound lean ground turkey

¼ teaspoon salt

1 teaspoon chili powder

1 teaspoon ground cumin

½ cup water

Fixings:

12 taco shells or 10 burrito tortillas*

½ cup sliced black olives

½ ripe avocado, sliced

1 cup finely chopped lettuce

1 large tomato, chopped

Kernels cut from 1 ear of corn, or 1 8-ounce can corn kernels or ½ frozen 10-ounce package of corn kernels

3 ounces Cheddar cheese, grated

1 cup salsa

*I like to use taco shells rather than burrito tortillas because the taco shells are made from whole grains and most burrito shells aren't—unless you get whole-wheat tortillas, which are available in health-food stores.

To make the beans
(if using canned beans, skip to step 4):

1. In a cooking pot, rinse and soak raw beans in 4 cups cold water for one hour.

2. Gently cook the beans in the water until tender—about 1 hour. Add more water if necessary.

3. Drain the beans, reserving the liquid.

4. Heat oil in a pan until fragrant. Add the onion and sauté for about 5 minutes. Add the pimento and continue sautéing for 5 more minutes.

5. Pour in the beans, and season with wine, salt, oregano, sugar, and chipotle pepper.

6. Simmer over medium heat until creamy, adding reserved liquid to reach a smooth, creamy consistency.

To make the rice:

1. In a saucepan, heat the oil. Add the garlic and onion. Sauté until the onion is transparent.

2. Add salt and chili powder and heat through for a minute.

3. Add rice and stir to coat. Cook about another 2 minutes.

4. Add water. Cover. Lower heat and cook until water is absorbed— about 40 minutes. Keep warm until serving time.

To make the ground turkey:

1. Heat a heavy frying pan over medium heat. Add the ground turkey and break it up with a wooden spoon.

2. Add salt, chili powder, and cumin. Stir to mix seasoning through.

3. Add ½ cup water. Cook until absorbed.

4. Cover and keep warm until ready for serving.

Heat the taco or burrito shells, cover them, and place them along with the beans, rice, ground turkey, and the rest of the fixings on the table and let everyone help themselves to the rest.

Nutritional information per serving:

Calories: 660 (35 percent from fat)   **Carbohydrates:** 76 grams
Cholesterol: 49 milligrams   **Fat:** 29 grams (saturated fat: 7 grams)
Fiber: 6 grams   **Protein:** 18 grams   **Sodium:** 1,104 milligrams

Tamale Pie

This is a terrific one-pot meal and quite attractive when placed in the center of the table, as the corn crust rises up over the filling.

YIELD: 6 SERVINGS

¼ pound ground turkey

½ cup texturized vegetable protein, reconstituted with ⅝ cup water (simply add the water to the TVP, and the TVP absorbs the water)

2 cloves garlic

¾ cup chopped green pepper

1 cup corn kernels

1 cup kidney beans

16 ounces tomato sauce (no salt added)

¼ cup sliced black olives

¼ cup salsa

2 teaspoons chili powder

1 cup yellow cornmeal

2½ cups water

Pinch salt

½ cup grated part-skim mozzarella cheese

1. Preheat the oven to 375°F.

2. In a nonstick frying pan, brown the ground turkey. Add the garlic, cook 2 minutes, then add the reconstituted soy protein. Add green peppers, corn, kidney beans, tomato sauce, olives, salsa, and chili powder. Pour mixture into a 10-inch x 10-inch baking pan or a 10-inch cast iron frying pan (make sure the handle is oven-safe).

3. In a saucepan, combine the water, cornmeal, and salt. Bring mixture to a boil until it thickens slightly. Spoon over top of meat and vegetable mixture.

4. Bake for 45 minutes. Remove from oven and sprinkle cheese on top. Return pan to oven and bake another 15 minutes.

Nutritional information per serving:

Calories: 355 (18 percent from fat) **Carbohydrates:** 60 grams
Cholesterol: 24 milligrams **Fat:** 7 grams **Fiber:** 6 grams
Protein: 17 grams **Sodium** 1,053 milligrams

Chicken/Tofu/Broccoli Stir-Fry

This recipe combines broccoli along with chicken, tofu, and brown rice to make a complete and satisfying dish. This meal is a good way to introduce the uninitiated family to tofu. As a mother, I've experienced frustration when I've worked hard to prepare a nutritious meal and was met by the groans and clenched jaws of young children who refused to eat anything "yucky." I had put so much time and energy into the preparation of the meal, and I couldn't even enjoy the fruits of my labor. This is a good way to get your family to try tofu with little resistance.

YIELD: 4 SERVINGS

2 cups water

1 cup brown rice

¾ cup low-sodium chicken broth

3 tablespoons soy sauce

¼ teaspoon ground ginger

¼ teaspoon garlic powder

2 teaspoons cornstarch

2 carrots cut in julienne strips

1½ cups broccoli flowerets

2 chicken cutlets, sliced thin on the diagonal

1 tablespoon sesame oil

2 or 3 sliced scallions

½ pound firm tofu, cubed

1. In a small pot, bring water to a boil. Add rice. Cook over low heat until all the water is absorbed. This should take about 40 minutes. (If your stovetop heat is difficult to modulate, a heat diffuser works well to ensure that brown rice cooks slowly enough to guarantee complete cooking.)

2. Pour the chicken broth and soy sauce in a small bowl. Add the ginger, garlic powder, and cornstarch. Stir well to mix. Set aside.

3. Fill a medium-sized pot with water and bring it to a boil. Add the carrots and broccoli. Cook 1 minute. Remove the vegetables with a slotted spoon and set them aside.

4. Put the sliced chicken in the boiling water. Stir. As soon as it turns from pink to white (less than 1 minute), remove the chicken.

5. In a large, heavy skillet, heat the sesame oil. Add the scallions. Cook 1 minute. Add the tofu and stir to mix. Add the par-cooked chicken and the vegetables. Remix the chicken broth mixture and add it to food in the skillet. Cook a few minutes to coat the chicken and tofu with the broth and spice mixture.

6. Serve over the rice.

Nutritional information per serving:

Calories: 392 (25 percent from fat)   **Carbohydrates:** 44 grams
Cholesterol: 33 milligrams   **Fat:** 11 grams   **Fiber:** 3.5 grams
Protein: 32 grams   **Sodium:** 1,110 milligrams

Soy It Up!

A good way to increase the phytochemical content of any dish in which chopped meat is used is to substitute some of the meat with texturized soy protein. Texturized soy protein is made from defatted soy flour. It is widely used as a meat extender or meat substitute. Archer Daniel's Midland Company owns the right to the name of Textured Vegetable Protein or TVP. It is also sold under the name soy nuggets. It is sold dried in granular and chunk style in natural food stores and through mail-order catalogs. When used as a meat substitute or extender, it is reconstituted with water and added in place of all or part of the meat used in recipes. It comes in handy for feeding the phytochemical-resistant diner. I've replaced about one-quarter of the ground turkey in recipes without anyone noticing. Ultimately, it's great for replacing meat altogether. It's also very inexpensive and needs no refrigeration or special storage.

Spicy Pasta with Artichoke Sauce

This delicious pasta dish is one of my favorites, and it is easy to make, since it calls for many ready-prepared ingredients. Try whipping up this one tonight.

YIELD: 4 SERVINGS

8 ounces any one-inch-size pasta (penne, rigatoni, or bow ties)

1 tablespoon olive oil

1 medium yellow onion, diced

1 tablespoon fresh garlic, minced

1 pound chopped fresh or canned tomatoes

1 cup sliced mushrooms

1 teaspoon dried basil

1 teaspoon dried oregano

Scant ¼ teaspoon cayenne pepper

¼ teaspoon freshly ground black pepper

1 14-ounce can artichoke hearts, quartered

2 tablespoons lemon juice

½ cup plus 2 tablespoons Parmesan cheese

1. Cook the pasta al dente according to package directions. Drain well and return the pasta to the pot.

2. While the pasta is cooking, sauté the olive oil in a large skillet. Add the onion and garlic. Cover and sweat the vegetables until the onions are transparent. Add tomatoes, mushrooms, basil, oregano, and cayenne and black pepper. Cook over medium-low heat for 10 to 15 minutes.

3. Add the artichokes and lemon juice. Cook for an additional 5 minutes. Reduce the heat to low.

4. Add the pasta to the skillet mixture and toss gently to mix. Add the Parmesan cheese. Toss gently and serve.

Nutritional information per serving:

Calories: 360   **Carbohydrates:** 62 milligrams   **Cholesterol:** 3.2 grams
Fat: 12 grams (30 percent of calories)   **Fiber:** 3.6 grams
Protein: 14 grams   **Sodium:** 322 milligrams

Just Desserts

Desserts may seem like an unlikely place to find phyto-chemicals, but they are actually the perfect way to boost your phytochemical intake. Here are a few tasty possibilities you can add to your menu.

New Wave Mighty Fine Chocolate Pudding

This pudding makes a nice dessert. The combination of soymilk with kuzu delivers a hefty dose of isoflavones.

YIELD: 4 SERVINGS

6 tablespoons kuzu powder*

2 cups chocolate flavored soymilk

2 teaspoons maple syrup

*You can pulverize the starch commonly found in health-food stores with a mortar and pestle or coffee grinder into a powder.

1. In a small bowl, mix the kuzu powder with 4 tablespoons of the soymilk until dissolved.

2. Put the remaining soymilk in a small saucepan over low heat. Stir in the kuzu mixture and maple syrup. Stir constantly until thickened.

3. Pour into 4 dessert cups and chill before serving.

Variation: During the holiday season, try using egg-nog-flavored soymilk.

Nutritional information per serving:

Calories: 107 (14 percent from fat) **Carbohydrates:** 19 grams
Cholesterol: 0 milligrams **Fat:** 1.2 grams **Fiber:** less than 1 gram
Protein: 5 grams **Sodium:** 47 grams

Sweet Maple Nuggets

Munch on a handful of these nuggets or sprinkle them on cereal, yogurt, or applesauce for a little crunch and a lot of nutrients.

YIELD: ½ CUP—ABOUT 4 SERVINGS

½ cup textured soy protein

1 tablespoon maple syrup

Microwave method:

Put the soy protein into a microwave-safe pie plate. Add the maple syrup, and stir to mix well. Spread it evenly across the plate. Microwave on high for about 3 minutes, stirring nearly every 20 seconds to avoid scorched spots. Nuggets are done when golden brown and only slightly sticky to the touch. Allow to cool, and then crumble it with your fingers.

Oven method:

Mix the soy protein and maple syrup, then spread evenly on a nonstick cookie sheet. Cook in a 300°F oven for about 6 minutes, stirring often. Watch carefully near the end. Bake 1 minute more if nuggets are sticky when cool.

Nutritional information per serving:

Calories: 54 (0 percent from fat) **Carbohydrates:** 9 grams
Cholesterol: 0 milligrams **Fat:** 0 grams **Fiber:** 2 grams
Protein: 7 grams **Sodium:** 3 milligrams

A Trifle Better Parfait

Your kids will love this fun, wholesome dessert.

YIELD: 4 SERVINGS

2 cups plain low-fat yogurt

1 tablespoon maple syrup

½ teaspoon vanilla extract

1 cup sliced fresh fruit

½ cup Maple Nuggets (see recipe on page 203)

1. In a small bowl, mix the yogurt, maple syrup, and the vanilla extract together. Set aside.

2. In drinking glasses or deep dessert dishes, layer the sliced fruit, yogurt mixture, and maple nuggets. Begin with the fruit and finish off with the yogurt topped with maple nuggets. Chill at least 1 hour and serve.

Nutritional information per serving:

Calories: 156 (10 percent from fat) **Carbohydrates:** 25 grams
Cholesterol: 6.7 milligrams **Fat:** 1.7 grams **Fiber:** less than 1 gram
Protein: 13 grams **Sodium:** 80 milligrams

Apple Crisp

This is a luscious dessert, perfect served warm on a crisp autumn day. Top it with a tablespoon of vanilla yogurt for an extra special touch.

YIELD: 6 SERVINGS

Filling:

4 cups sliced cooking apples

2 tablespoons flour

2 tablespoons maple syrup

2 tablespoons honey

½ teaspoon cinnamon

Topping:

⅓ cup dry textured soy protein

½ cup whole oats

2 tablespoons maple syrup

2 tablespoons honey

¼ teaspoon cinnamon

2 tablespoons melted butter

1. Preheat the oven to 350°F.

2. Put the apples in a medium bowl. Combine the flour, maple syrup, honey, and cinnamon and pour over the fruit. Stir well to coat the fruit. Place the mixture into an 8- or 9-inch square baking dish.

3. Combine all topping ingredients except the butter in a small mixing bowl. Add the melted butter and stir to combine well. Sprinkle the topping over the fruit mixture.

4. Bake for 45 minutes until filling bubbles around the edges. Serve either warm or cold.

Nutritional information per serving:

Calories: 201 (22 percent from fat) **Carbohydrates:** 37 grams
Cholesterol: 10.8 milligrams **Fat:** 5 grams **Fiber:** 2.8 grams
Protein: 6.8 grams **Sodium:** 127 milligrams

Conclusion

 For the past several years, while researching and writing this book, I also have worked as a traditional dietitian in a community hospital. Daily, I find more and more research pointing to the fact that nutrition is the first step to maintaining good health. Plant foods have the ability to play a vital role in the health-care process. However, I am constantly frustrated by the fact that this information is not being put to use in our health-care institutions. Even in the finest of our health-care facilities, the emphasis on food as a healing tool is less than it could be.

As a society, we do not take adequate advantage of the medicinal uses of food. A lot of time and newspaper ink is spent in the debate about the escalating costs of health care, but there is a proven, inexpensive way of defraying some of these costs right in our midst that is largely ignored by the medical community. Nutrition therapy is the least expensive and most risk-free health-care option. If we truly want to reduce health-care costs, we must integrate respect for nutrition into our society. If we teach people to take care of themselves while they are well, there will be less sickness. Our concept of what conventional medicine is needs to be changed. Why is nutritional healing considered unconventional medicine, while the pumping of toxins into one's bloodstream is considered conventional? As often happens, my research has raised as many new questions for me as it has raised answers.

The members of the medical profession must be convinced to find out the truth for themselves. If aggressive nutrition therapy could be integrated into the traditional hospital setting, the length of hospital stays as well as health-care costs would be reduced. This would truly be integrative medicine—the blending of "unconventional" medicine with "conventional" medicine. I am not advocating doing away with the current system of medicine, only refining it and making it even better.

The concept of making dietary changes to alter the disease process is not new. For centuries, people have been improving their health through diet. What is new is the discovery of the way in which specific substances in plant foods assist the body in fending off disease. We can take this information and use it wisely by incorporating it into our health-care practice. Using phytochemicals in plant foods to fight disease is cost-efficient and self-empowering. The challenge we are now faced with is finding as many opportunities as we can to incorporate phytochemical-rich foods into our lives.

References

Chapter 1—What Are Phytochemicals?

American Dietetic Association, Position Paper: *Phytochemicals and Functional Foods. Journal of the American Dietetic Association, 95(4)* (April 1995).

Bradlow, H. Leon. Interview, July 21, 1995, at Strang Cornell Research Labs, NYC, N.Y.

California Raisin Marketing Board. "Snack on Raisins for Antioxidants." *Raisin Renaissance* (Summer 1999).

Craig, W.J. "Phytochemicals: Guardians of Our Health." *Journal of the American Dietetic Association* (1997):S199–S204.

DiMasco, P., "Antioxidant Defense Systems: The Role of Carotenoids, Tocopherols and Thiols." *American Journal of Clinical Nutrition* 53 (1991):194S–200S.

Elson, Charles. Personal communication, April 22, 1998. University of Wisconsin at Madison.

LaChance, Paul. "Nutraceuticals." Address to the New York State Dietetic Association, April 24, 1998.

McBride, J. "Plant Pigments: Paint a Rainbow of Antioxidants." *Agricultural Research Magazine,* April 1996.

Pinto, John. "Phytochemicals and Cancer." Presentation to the Mid-Hudson Dietetic Association, April 8, 1998.

Prior, R.L., et al. "Can Foods Forestall Aging?" *Agricultural Research Magazine,* February 1999.

Steinmetz, K.A., Potter J.D. "Vegetables, Fruit and Cancer II: Mechanisms." *Cancer, Causes and Control* 2 (1991): 427–442.

Wattenberg, L.W. "Inhibition of Carcinogenesis of Minor Dietary Constituents." *Cancer Research* 52 (April 1, 1992) (supplement): 2085s–2091s.

Chapter 2—The History of Phytochemicals

American Dietetic Association Position Paper: *Phytochemicals and Functional Foods. Journal of the American Dietetic Association* 95(4) (April 1995): 493–496.

American Institute of Cancer Research, World Cancer Research Fund, *Food, Nutrition and the Prevention of Cancer: A Global Perspective,* 1997.

Bradlow, H. Leon. Interview, July 21, 1995, at Strang Cornell Research Labs, NYC, N.Y.

Giovannucci, A.A., et al. "Intake of Carotenoids and Retinol in Relation to Risk of Prostate Cancer," *Journal of the National Cancer Institute* 87(23) (December 6, 1995).

Greenwald, P. "Scientific America." *Chemoprevention of Cancer* (September 1996): 96.

Michnovicz, J.J., Bradlow, H.L., "Altered Estrogen Metabolism and Excretion in Humans Following Consumption of Indole-3-Carbinol." *Nutrition Cancer* 16 (1991): 59–66.

Stacey, M. "The Rice and Fall of Kilmer McCully." *The New York Times Magazine* (August 10, 1997): 25.

Steinmetz, K.A., Potter, J.D. "Vegetables, Fruit and Cancer: II Mechanisms." *Cancer, Causes and Control* 2 (1991): 427–442.

Tiwari, R.K., et al. "Selective Responsiveness of Human Breast Cancer Cells to Indole-3-Carbinol, a Chemopreventive Agent." *Journal of the National Cancer Institute (86)*2 (1994): 126–131.

Wallis, C. "Curing Cancer—The Hype and the Hope," *Time Magazine* (May 18, 1998): 38–50.

Chapter 3—Phytochemicals from A to Z

Agarwal, R., et al. "Inhibitory Effect of Silymarin, an Anti-Hepatoxic Flavonoid, on 12-o-tetradecanoylphorbol-13-acetate Induced Epidermal Ornitine Carboxylase Activity and Mrna in Sencar Mice." *Carcinogenesis,* 15(6) (1994): 1099–1103.

Ameer, B., Weintraub, R.A. "Drug Interactions with Grapefruit Juice." *Clinical Pharmakinetics* 33(2) (1997): 103–21.

American Diabetes Association, *Maximizing the Role of Nutrition in Diabetes Management,* 1994.

American Institute for Cancer Research. Newsletter, Winter 1997, Issue #54.

American Institute for Cancer Research, World Cancer Research Fund, *Food, Nutrition and the Prevention of Cancer: A Global Perspective*, 1997.

Anderson J.W., Johnstone, B.M., Cook-Newell, M.E. "Meta-Analysis of the Effects of Soy Protein Intake on Serum Lipids." *The New England Journal of Medicine* (August 3, 1995): 276–282.

Aoki, T., Miyakoshi, H., Horikawa, Y., Usuda, Y. *Augmenting Agents in Cancer Therapy.* "Staphage lysate and Lentinan as immunoodulators and/or immunopotentiators in clinic and experimental systems." New York: Raven Press, pp.101–112 (1981).

"Ask Us." *Diabetes Forecast* (September 1997): 57.

Barnes, S., Kim, H. "Soy Isoflavones, Estrogens and Growth Factor Signaling." *The Soy Connection* 6(2), Spring 1998.

Beckstrom-Sternberg, Stephen M., Duke, James A. "The Phytochemical Data Base" *http//probe.nalusda.gov.8300/cgi-bin/browse/phytochem db*, July 1994.

Berges, R.R., et al. "Randomised, Placebo-Controlled, Double-Blind Clinical Trial of B-Sitosterol in Patients with Benign Prostatic Hyperplasia." *The Lancet,* Vol. 345, June 17, 1995, 1529–1532.

Block, E. "The Chemistry of Garlic and Onions." *Scientific American,* 1985:252, 114–119.

Bradlow, H. Leon. Personal Communication, July 21, 1995, at Strang Cornell Research Labs, NYC, N.Y.

———. Personal Communication, April 22, 1998, Strang Cornell Research Center for Breast Cancer Research.

Brody, J. "A New Look at an Ancient Remedy: Celery." *New York Times,* June 9, 1992, page C-3.

Caragay, A.B. "Cancer-Preventive Foods and Ingredients." *Food Technology,* April 1992, 65–68.

Chihara, G., et al. "Anti-tumor and Metastasis—Inhibitory Activities of Lentinan as an Immunomodulator." *Cancer Detection and Prevention.* Supplement (1987) 1, pp. 423.

Clarke, R. Dietary Phytochemicals in Cancer Prevention and Treatment. Session III. "Estrogen, Phytoestrogens and Breast Cancer." AICR Annual Research Conference. August 31, 1995.

Clarke, R., et al. *Advances in Experimental Medicine and Biology.* "Estrogens, Phytoestrogens and Breast Cancer" "Dietary Phytochemicals in Cancer Prevention and Treatment." American Institute for Cancer Research, Volume 401.

Columbia University. Notes and Handouts from the meeting "Botanical Medicine in Modern Clinical Practice." Columbia University College of Physicians and Surgeons, May 13–17, 1996. Speaker: Dr. Andrew Weil.

Craig, W.J. "Phytochemicals: Guardians of Our Health." *Journal of the American Dietetic Association,* 1997 (Supplement 2): S199–S204.

Crowell, P.L., Ayoubi, S.A., Burke, Y.D. "Antitumorgeric Effects of Limonene and Perillyl Alcohol Against Pancreatic and Breast Cancer." *Dietary Phytochemicals in Cancer Prevention and Treatment.* New York: Plenum Press, 1996.

Dalais, F.S. "Soy and Menopause." *The Soy Connection,* Vol. 5, No. 4, Fall 1997.

DiMasco, P., Murphy, M.E., Sies, H. "Antioxidant Defense Systems: The Role of Carotenoids, Tocopherols and Thiols." *American Journal of Clinical Nutrition* 53 (1991):194S–200S.

Duke, James. Phone, Personal Communication, January 30, 1998.

Elson, C.E., Yu, S.G. "The Chemoprevention of Cancer by Mevalonate-Derived Constituents of Fruits and Vegetables." *American Institute of Nutrition* (Dec. 1993): 607–614.

Elson, Charles. Personal communication, April 22, 1998. University of Wisconsin at Madison.

Erdman J.W., Bierer T.L., Gugger E.T. "Absorption and Transport of Carotenoids in Human Health." *Annals of the New York Academy of Sciences 691* (December 31, 1993).

Erdman, J.W., Potter S.M. "Soy and Bone Health," *The Soy Connection,* Spring 1997.

Fiala, E.S., Reddy, B.S., Weisburger, J.H. "Naturally Occurring Anticarcinogenic Substances in Foodstuffs." *Annual Reviews in Nutrition* 5 (1985): 295–321.

Giovannucci, A.A., et al. "Intake of Carotenoids and Retinol in Relation to Risk of Prostate Cancer." *Journal of the National Cancer Institute* 87(23) (Dec. 6, 1995).

"Grapefruit Can Interact with Medications." *Harvard Heart Letter,* April 1999.

Hecht, S.S., Personal communication, American Health Foundation, Valhalla, N.Y.

Hecht, S.S., et al. "Effects of Watercress Consumption on Metabolism of a Tobacco-specific Lung Carcinogen in Smokers." *Cancer Epidemiology, Biomarkers and Prevention* 4 (December 1995): 877–884.

Hunt, Sara, M., Groff, James L. *Advanced Nutrition and Human Metabolism.* West Publishing Company, 1990.

Indiana Soybean Development Council. *U.S. 1997 Soyfoods Directory.*

Ip, C., Lisk, D.J. "Enrichment with Selenium of Allium Vegetables for Cancer Prevention," *Carcinogenesis* 15(9) (1994): 1851–1885.

Jang, M. "Cancer Chemopreventive Activity of Resveratrol, a Natural Product Derived from Grapes," *Science* 275 (January 10, 1997).

Jankun, J., et al. "Why Drinking Green Tea Could Prevent Cancer," *Nature* 387 (1997): 561.

Kaufman, P.B. "A Comparative Survey of Leguminous Plants as Sources of the Isoflavones, Genistein and Daidzein: Implications for Human Nutrition and Health." *The Journal of Alternative and Complementary Medicine* 3(1) (1997): 7–12.

Kelly, G.S. "Bromelain: A Literature Review and Discussion of Its Therapeutic Applications." *Alternative Medicine Reviews1(4)* (1996).

Kennedy A.R., et al. "Suppression of Carcinogenesis in the Intestines of Min Mice in the Soybean Derived Bowman-Birk Inhibitor." *Cancer Research* 56 (1996): 679.

Kensler, T.W., et al. "Mechanism of Protection Against Aflatoxin Tumorgenicity in Rate Fed 5-(2-Pyranzinyl)-4-methyl-1,2-dithiol-3-thione (Oltipraz) and Related 1,2 Dithiol-3-thiones and 1,2-Dithiolethiones." *Cancer Research* 47 (August 15, 1987): 4271–4277.

Khechai, F. "Effect of Advanced Glycation End Product-modified Albumin on Tissue Factor Expression by Monocytes. Role of Oxidant Stress and Protein Tyrosine Kinase Activation." *Arteriosclerosis, Thrombosis, & Vascular Biology* 17(11) (1997): 2885–2890.

Knight, D.C., Eden, J.A. "A Review of the Clinical Effects of Phytoestrogens." *Obstetrics and Gynecology* 87(5), Part 2 (May 1996).

Krause, Mahan. *Food Nutrition and Diet Therapy,* 7th ed. W.B. Saunders and Co.

Kurowska, E.M. "Soy and Reduced Risk of Cardiovascular Disease." *The Soy Connection* 5(3) (Summer 1997).

Leaf, A., Weber, P.C. "Cardiovascular Effects of N-3 Fatty Acids." *New England Journal of Medicine* 318(9) (March 3, 1988).

Michnovicz J.J., Bradlow, H.L. "Altered Estrogen Metabolism and Excretion in Humans Following Consumption of Indole-3-Carbinol." *Nutrition Cancer* 16 (1991): 59–66.

Mitchell, P. "Grapefruit Juice Found to Cause Havoc." *The Lancet* 353 (April 17, 1999).

Morse, M.A., et al. "Inhibition of 4(methylnitrosamino)-1-3pyridyl)-1 butanone induced DNA Adduct Formation and Tumorgenicity in the Lung of F344 Rats by Dietary Phenethyl Isothiocynate." *Cancer Research* 49 (February 1989): 549–553.

Muktar, H., Katiyar, S.K., Agarwal, R. "Cancer Chemoprevention by Green Tea Components. Diet and Cancer: Markers Prevention and Treatment." Plenum Press, New York, 1994.

Murkies, A.L., et al. "Dietary Flour Supplementation Decreases Post-Menopausal Hot Flushes: Effect of Soy and Wheat." *Maturitas* 3 (April 21, 1995): 189–195.

Pawlak, Laura, *A Perfect Ten: Phyto "New-Trients" Against Cancers.* Biomed General Corp., Emeryville, California, 1998.

Potter, S.M. "Overview of Proposed Mechanisms for the Hypocholesterolemic Effect of Soy." *Journal of Nutrition* 125 (1995): 606S–611S.

Pronsky, Z.M. *Powers and Moore's Food Medications Interactions,* 9th ed.

Proulx W., Weaver, C.M. "Calcium Absorption from Plants." *The Soy Connection* 2 (2).

Rose, D.R. "Dietary Fatty Acids and Cancer." *American Journal of Clinical Nutrition* 66 (1997) (Supplement): 998S–1003S.

Ross Products Division, Abbott Laboratories, *What You Should Know About FOS,* October 1997.

Salmi, H.A., Sarna, S. "Effect of Silymarin on Chemical, Functional and Morphological Alterations of the Liver." *Scandinavian Journal of Gastroenterology,* 1982, 17, 517–521.

Schardt D., Leibman B. "Garlic vs. Garlic." *Center for Science in the Public Interest, Nutrition Action Health Letter* 22(6) (July/August 1995).

Schardt, David. "Phytochemicals—Plants Against Cancer." *Nutrition Action Health Letter,* Center for Science in the Public Interest, Vol. 21. No. 3, April 1994.

Schelp F.P., Pongpaew, P. "Protection Against Cancer Through Nutritionally Induced Increase of Endogenous Proteinase Inhibitors-A Hypothesis." *International Journal of Epidemiology* 17(2) (1998).

Schulze, J., Malone, A. Richter, E. "Intestional Metabolism of 4-(methylnitrosamino-1-(3-pyridyl)1-butanone in Rats: Sex-Difference, Inductibility and Inhibition by Phenethylisothiocyanate." *Carcinogenesis* 16 (1995): 1733–1740.

Seddon, J.M., et al., "Dietary Carotenoids, Vitamin A, C, and E and Advanced Age-related Macular Degeneration." *Journal of the American Medical Association* 2723 (18) (November 9, 1994): 1413–1420.

Simopoulos, A.P. "Common Purslane: A Source of Omega-3 Fatty Acids and Antioxidants." *Journal of the American College of Nutrition,* (H51)11(4) (August 1992): 374–382.

Steinmetz, K.A., Potter, J.D. "Vegetables, Fruit and Cancer: II Mechanisms." *Cancer, Causes and Control* 2 (1991): 427–442.

Sugiyama, K., et al. "Dietary Eritadenine Modifies Plasma Phosphatidylcholine Molecular Species Profile in Rats Fed Different Types of Fat." *Journal of Nutrition* 127 (1997): 593–599.

Tiwari, R.K., et al. "Selective Responsiveness of Human Breast Cancer to Indole-3-Carbinol, a Chemopreventive Agent." *Journal of the National Cancer Insitute* 86(2) (1994):126–131.

Wang, H., Murphy P. "Isoflavone Content in Commercial Soybean Foods." *Journal of Agricultural Food Chemists* 42 (1994): 1666–1673.

Wattenberg, L.W. "Inhibition of Carcinogenesis of Minor Dietary Constituents." *Cancer Research* 52 (April 1, 1992) (Supplement): 2085s—2091s.

Weed, S.S. Menopausal Years, The Wise Woman Way. Woodstock, New York: Ash Tree Publishing, 1992.

"When Grapefruit Juice and Drugs Mix." *Tufts University Health and Nutrition Letter,* March 1997.

Whitney, E.N., Hamilton, E.M.N. *Understanding Nutrition.* West Publishing Co., 1987.

Women's Health Advocate Newsletter.

Yu, Sha, et al. "Anti-Tumor Activity of the Crude Saponins Obtained from Asparagus." *Cancer Letters* 104 (1996): 31–36.

Zheng, G., Kenney, P.M., Zhang, J., Lam, L.K.T. "Chemoprevention of Benzo(a)pyrene-Induced Forestomach Cancer in Mice by Natural Phtalides from Celery Seed Oil." *Nutrition Cancer* 19 (1993): 77–86.

Zheng, G.Q., Kenney, P.M., Lam, L.K.T. "Anethofuran, Carvone and Limonene: Potential Cancer Chemopreventive Agents from Dill Weed Oil and Caraway Oil." *Planta Medica* 58 (1992).

Chapter 4—The Most Powerful Foods

Agarwal, R., et al. "Inhibitory Effect of Silymarin, an Anti-Hepatotoxic Flavonoid, on 12-O-tetraecanoylphorbol-13-acetate Induced Epidermal Ornithine Carboxylase Activity and mRNA in Senccar Mice." *Carcinogenesis* 15(6) (1994): 1099–1103.

Ballister, B. *Fruit and Vegetable Stand.* Woodstock, New York: Overlook Press, 1985.

Barnes, S., Kim, H., "Soy Isoflavones, Estrogens and Growth Factor Signaling." *The Soy Connection* 6 (2) (Spring 1998).

Beckstrom-Sternberg, Stephen M., James A. Duke. "The Phytochemical Database." *http//probe.nalusda .gov.8300/cgi-bin/browse/phytochem d* July 1994.

Block, E. "The Chemistry of Garlic and Onions." *Scientific American* 252 (1985): 114–119.

Brown, L, et al. "Cholesterol-Lowering Effects of Dietary Fiber: A Meta-Analysis." *American Journal of Clinical Nutrition* 69 (1999): 30–42.

Caragay, A.B. "Cancer-Preventive Foods and Ingredients." *Food Technology* (April 1992): 65–68.

Columbia University. Notes and Handouts from the meeting "Botanical Medicine in Modern Clinical Practice." Columbia University College of Physicians and Surgeons, May 13–17, 1996. Speaker, Dr. Andrew Weil. November 6, 1997.

Craig, W.J. "Phytochemicals: Guardians of Our Health," *Journal of the American Dietetic Association* (1997) (supplement 2): S199–S204.

Crowell, P.L., Ayoubi, S.A., Burke, Y.D. "Antitumorgenic Effects of Limonene and Perillyl Alcohol Against Pancreatic and Breast Cancer." *Dietary Phytochemicals in Cancer Prevention and Treatment.* Pleneum Press, New York, 1996.

Cunnane, S.C., et al. "High Alpha Linolenic Acid Flaxseed: Some Nutritional Properties in Humans." *British Journal of Nutrition* 69 (1993): 443–453.

Erdman, J.W., Bierer, T.L., Gugger, E.T., "Absorption and Transport of Carotenoids: Carotenoids in Human Health." *Annals of the New York Academy of Sciences* 691 (Dec. 31, 1993).

Fahey, J.W., et al. "Broccoli Sprouts; An Exceptionally Rich Source of Inducers of Enzymes that Protect Against Chemical Carcinogen." *Proceedings of the National Academy of Science* 94(9) (September 1997): 10367–10372.

Gold Medal Cook Book. Minneapolis, MN: Washburn-Crosby Co., 1904.

Goldbeck, D.N. *American Whole Foods Cuisine.* New American Library, 1983.

Hecht S.S., et al. "Effects of Watercress Consumption on Metabolism of a Tobacco-specific Lung Carcinogen in Smokers." *Cancer Epidemiology, Biomarkers and Prevention* 4 (December 1985): 877–884.

Hunter, Julie. "Stalking Greens, Potherbs and Shoots." *Countryside & Small Stock Journal* 82(3) (1998): 59.

Hylton, W.M., ed. *The Rodale Herb Book.* Hylton Rodale Press, 1976.

Jang, M., et al. "Cancer Chemopreventive Activity of Resveratrol, a Natural Product Derived from Grapes." *Science* 275 (Jan. 10, 1997).

Kaufman, P.B., et al. "A Comparative Survey of Leguminous Plants as Sources of the Isoflavones, Genistein and Daidzein: Implications for Human Nutrition and Health." *The Journal of Alternative and Complementary Medicine* 3(1) (1997): 7–12.

Knight, D.C., Eden, J.A. "A Review of the Clinical Effects of Phytoestrogens," *Obstetrics and Gynecology* 87(5) Part 2 (May 1996).

Kryger, Abraham. Personal Research.

Mangels, A.R., et al. "Carotenoid Content of Fruits and Vegetables: An Evaluation of Analytic Data." *Journal of the American Dietetic Association* 93 (1993): 284–296.

Messina, M. "Soy Shows Promise in Slowing Prostate Cancer Rate of Growth." *The Soy Connection*, Volume 6, November 4, Fall 1998.

Mindell, E. *Earl Mindell's Soy Miracle*. Fireside Books, 1995.

Muktar, H., Katiyar, S.K., Agarwal, R. "Cancer Chemoprevention by Green Tea Components." In *Diet and Cancer: Markers Prevention and Treatment*. New York: Plenum Press, 1994.

Pawlak, Laura. *A Perfect Ten: Phyto "New-Trients" Against Cancers*. Biomed General Corp.: Emeryville, California, 1998.

Pronsky, Z.M. *Powers and Moore's Food Medications Interactions*, 9th ed.

Proulx, W., Weaver, C.M. "Calcium Absorption from Plants," *The Soy Connection* Volume 2, Number 2.

Research presented at the American Chemical Society Meeting, September 1997.

Ross Products Division, Abbott Laboratories, *What You Should Know About FOS*.

Salmi, H.A., Sarna, S. "Effect of Silymarin on Chemical, Functional and Morphological Alterations of the Liver." *Scandinavian Journal of Gastroenterology* 17 (1982): 517–521.

Schardt, David. "Phytochemicals—Plants Against Cancer." *Nutrition Action Health Letter*, Center for Science in the Public Interest 21(3) (April 1994).

Simopoulos, A.P. "Common Purslane: A Source of Omega-3 Fatty Acids and Antioxidants." *Journal of the American College of Nutrition* (H51)11(4) (August 1992): 374–82.

Stein, Jess, ed. *The Random House Dictionary of the English Language*. New York, 1968.

Steinmetz, K.A., et al. "Vegetables, Fruit and Colon Cancer in the Iowa's Women's Health Study." *The American Journal of Epidemiology* 139(1) (1994).

Steinmetz, K.A., Potter, J.D. "Vegetables, Fruit and Cancer: II Mechanisms." *Cancer, Causes and Control* 2 (1991): 427–442.

Thoreau, Henry David. *Walden or Life in the Woods*. Mount Vernon, New York: Peter Pauper Press.

The Tomato Research Council. Notes from International Symposium on the Role of Lycopene and Tomato Products in Disease Prevention. March 3, 1997.

U.S. Soyfoods Directory 1998. *Indiana Soybean Board, Lebanon, Indiana*.

USDA Nutrient Database for Standard Reference.

Visoli, F., Galli, C. "The Effect of Minor Constituents of Olive Oil on Cardiovascular Disease: New Findings." *Nutrition Reviews* 56(5) (1998): 142–147.

Whitney, E.N., Hamilton, E.M.N. *Understanding Nutrition*. West Publishing Co., 1987.

Woman's Day Encyclopedia of Cookery.

Yu, Sha, et al., "Anti-Tumor Activity of the Crude Saponins Obtained from Asparagus." *Cancer Letters* 104 (1996): 31–36.

Zheng, G., et al. "Chemoprevention of Benzo(a)pyrene-Induced Forestomach Cancer in Mice by Natural Phthalides from Celery Seed Oil." *Nutrition Cancer* 19 (1993): 77–86.

Chapter 5—Phytochemical Supplements

Fischer, U.F., Carstens, R. "The Real World of Phytochemicals (II): Loss of Phytonutrient Content in Juicing," Poster Abstract #61. Dietary Phytochemicals in Cancer Prevention and Treatment. 1995 Research Conference.

"Good News on Herb Supplements: Label's Ingredients Usually Accurate." *Investors Business Daily,* November 15, 1999, p. A-2.

Leiberman, Shari. *The Real Vitamin and Mineral Book.* Garden City Park, N.Y.: Avery Publishing Group, Inc., 1997.

Tastebud, Dr. "Ask Dr. Tastebud." *Nutrition Action Health Letter,* The Center for Science in the Public Interest, July/August 1998, page 14.

"Veggies in a Pill." *Women's Health Advocate Newsletter,* June 1998 5(4): 1–2, 8.

Chapter 6—The Basic Healthy Diet

Franz, M. "Eat Well, Feel Well." 1993, Pfizer, Inc.

http://www.fda.gov.

http://www.usda.gov.fcs/cnpp.

Mood, Mind & Appetite, Conference Presentor M. Freedman—sponsored by INR/Biomed Corp.

PART TWO—CONDITIONS TREATABLE WITH PHYTOCHEMICALS

Age-Related Macular Degeneration

International Food Information Council. "Food for Thought II." *Report of Diet, Nutrition and Food Safety,* February 1998.

Mares-Perlman, J.A., et al. "Serum Anti-oxidants and Age-Related Macular Degeneration in a Population-Based Case Control Study." *Archives of Opthalmology* 113 (Dec. 1995).

Seddon, J.M., et al. "Dietary Carotenoids, Vitamin A, C, and E and Advanced age-related Macular Degeneration," *Journal of the American Medical Association,* 2723(18) (November 9, 1994): 1413–1420.

www.macular.org, November 18, 1998.

Benign Hyperplasia of the Prostate

Beckstrom-Sternberg, Stephen M., Duke, James A. "The Phytochemical Data base." *http//probe.nalusda.gov.8300/cgi-bin/browse/phytochem db* (ACEDB version 4.3 date version), July 1994.

Berges, R.R., et al. "The B-Sitosterol Study Group Randomised, Placebo-Controlled, Double Blind Clinical Trial of B-sitosterol in Patients with Benign Prostatic Hyperplasia." *Lancet* 345 (1995): 1529–1532.

Columbia University. Notes and Handouts from the meeting "Botanical Medicine in Modern Clinical Practice." Columbia University College of Physicians and Surgeons, May 13–17, 1996, Speaker: Dr. Andrew Weil.

Oesterling, J.E. "Benign Prostatic Hyperplasia Medical and Minimally Invasive Treatment." *New England Journal of Medicine* 332(2) (Jan. 12, 1995).

Cancer

Agarwal, R., et al. "Inhibitory Effect of Silymarin, an Anti-Hepatotoxic Flavonoid, on 12-O-tetraecanoylphorbol-13-acetate Induced Epidermal Ornithine Carboxylase Activity and mRNA in Senccar Mice." *Carcinogenesis* 15(6) (1994): 1099–1103.

Carter, J.P., et al. "Hypothesis: Dietary Management May Improve Survival from Nutritionally Linked Cancers Based on Analysis of Representative Cases." *Journal of the American College of Nutrition* 12(3) (1993): 209–226.

Craig, W.J., "Phytochemicals: Guardians of Our Health." *Journal of the American Dietetic Association* (1997) (supplement 2): S199–S204.

Crowell, P.L., Ayoubi, S.A., Burke, Y.D. "Antitumorgenic Effects of Limonene and Perillyl Alcohol Against Pancreatic and Breast Cancer." *Dietary Phytochemicals in Cancer Prevention and Treatment.* New York: Pleneum Press, 1996.

"Dietary Factors." *Cancer Causes and Control* 7 (1996): S7–S9.

Djuric, Z., et al. "Oxidative DNA Damage Levels in Blood from Women at High Risk for Breast Cancer Are Associated with Dietary Intakes of Meats, Vegetables, and Fruits." *Journal of the American Dietetic Association* 98 (1998): 524–528.

LaFord. "Cancer, the Outlaw Cell." *Articles in Chemistry,* 1977, Vol. 50.

Messina, M. "Soy Shows Promise in Slowing Prostate Cancer Rate of Growth." *The Soy Connection,* Vol. 6, November 4, 1998.

Nash, M. "Stopping a Killer in Its Track." *Time Magazine,* April 25, 1994.

Pawlak, Laura. *A Perfect Ten: Phyto "New-Trients" Against Cancers.* Emeryville, Calif.: Biomed General Corp., 1998.

Rose, D.P., Hatala, M.A. "Dietary Fatty Acids and Breast Cancer Invasion and Metastasis." *Nutrition Cancer* 21(2) (1994): 103–111.

Salmi, B.A., Sarna, S. "Effect of Silymarin on Chemical, Functional and Morphological Alterations of the Liver." *Scandinavian Journal of Gastroenterology* 17 (1982): 517–521.

Uckun, F.M., et al. "Biotherapy of B-Cell Precursor Leukemia by Targeting Genistien to CD-19 Associated Tyrosine Kinases." *Science* 267 (Feb. 10, 1995).

Wattenberg, L.W. "Inhibition of Carcinogenesis of Minor Dietary Constituents." *Cancer Research* 52 (April 1, 1992) (Supplement): 2085s–2091s.

Yu, Sha, et. al. "Anti-Tumor Activity of the Crude Saponins Obtained from Asparagus" *Cancer Letters* 104 (1996): 31–36.

Candida

Beckstrom-Sternberg, Stephen, M., Duke, James A. The Phytochemical Data base. *http//probe.nalusda.gov.8300/cgi-bin/browse/phytochemdb* (ACEDB version 4.3 date version), July 1994.

Elmer, G.W., Surawicz, C.M., McFarland, L.V. "Biotherapeutic Agents," *Journal of the American Medical Association,* March 20, 1996.

Mandell, Douglas and Bennett. *Principles and Practice of Infectious Diseases.* Churchill Livingstone, 1995.

Ross Products Division, Abbott Laboratories, *What You Should Know About FOS.*

Spiegel, J.E., et al. "Safety and Benefits of Fructooligosaccharides as Food Ingredients." *Food Technology,* January 1994.

Cardiovascular Disease

Adler, A.J., Holub, B.J. "Effect of Garlic and Fish-oil Supplementation on Serum Lipid and Lipoprotein Concentrations in Hypercholesterolemic Men." *American Journal of Clinical Nutrition* 65 (1997): 445–450.

American Heart Association Web Site *www.aha.org.*

Anderson, J.W., Johnstone, B.M., Cook-Newell, M.E. "Meta-Analysis of the Effects of Soy Protein Intake on Serum Lipids." *New England Journal of Medicine* 333 (1993): 276–282.

Block, E. "The Chemistry of Garlic and Onions." *Scientific American* 252 (1985): 114–119.

Columbia University. Notes and Handouts from the meeting "Botanical Medicine in Modern Clinical Practice." Columbia University College of Physicians and Surgeons, May 13–17, 1996. Speaker: Dr. Andrew Weil.

Craig, W.J. "Phytochemicals: Guardians of Our Health." *Journal of the American Dietetic Association* (1997) (Supplement 2): S199–S204.

Cunnane, S.C., et al. "High Alpha Linolenic Acid Flaxseed: Some Nutritional Properties in Humans." *British Journal of Nutrition* 69 (1993): 443–453.

Folts, John D. Presented at a conference of the American College of Cardiology.

Imai, K., Nakachi, K. "Cross Sectional Study of Effects of Drinking Green Tea on Cardiovascular and Liver Disease" *British Medical Journal* 310 (March 18, 1995): 693–696.

Noble, H.B. "A Handful of Nuts and a Healthier Heart." *New York Times,* November 17, 1998.

"Phytochemicals: Drugstore in a Salad." *Consumer Reports on Health* 12 (December 1995): 133–135.

Prasad, K.N., et al. "High Doses of Multiple Antioxidant Vitamins: Essential Ingredients in Improving the Efficacy of Standard Cancer Therapy." *Journal of the American College of Nutrition* 18(1) (1999): 13–25.

Research presented at the American Chemical Society Meeting, September 1997.

Rimm, et al. "Folate and Vitamin B-6 Status from Diet and Supplements in Relation of Risk in Coronary Heart Disease Among Women." *Journal of the American Medical Association* 279(5) (1998): 359–364.

U.S. 1997 Soyfoods Directory. Published by the Indiana Development Soybean Council.

Diabetes

Anderson, James, et al. "Effects of Psylllium on Glucose and Serum Lipid Response in Men with Type 2 Diabetes and Hypercholesterolemia." *American Journal of Clinical Nutrition* 70 (1999): 466–473.

Anderson, R.A. "Chromium, Glucose Intolerance and Diabetes." *Journal of the American College of Nutrition* 17(6) (December 1998): 548–555.

Cunnane S.C., et al. "High Alpha Linolenic Acid Flaxseed: Some Nutritional Properties in Humans." *British Journal of Nutrition* 69 (1993): 443–453.

Deboles Company. Private communication, November 16, 1998.

Garg, Abhimanyu. "High Monunsaturated-Fat Diets for Patients with Diabetes Mellitus: A Meta-Analysis." *American Journal of Clinical Nutrition* 67 (1998) (Supplement): 577S–582S.

Khechai, F., et al. "Effect of Advanced Glycation End Product-Modified Albumin on Tissue Factor Expression by Monocytes. Role of Oxidant Stress and Protein Tyrosine Kinase Activation." *Arteriosclerosis, Thrombosis, & Vascular Biology*, 17(11) (November 1997): 2885–2890.

Maximizing the Role of Nutrition in Diabetes Management. American Diabetes Association, 1994.

Messina, Mark & Virginia. "Diet vs. Diabetes, Lean on the Bean Dietary Factors." *Cancer Causes and Control* 7 (1996): 57–59.

Mooradian, A.D., et al. "Selected Vitamins and Minerals in Diabetes." *Diabetes Care* 17(5) (May 1994): 464–479.

Ross Products Division, Abbott Laboratories. *What You Should Know About FOS.*

Rumessen, J. et al. "Fructans of Jerusalem Artichokes: Intestinal Transport, Absorption, Fermentation and Influence on Blood Glucose, Insulin and C-peptide Responses in Healthy Subjects." *American Journal for Clinical Nutrition* 52 (1990): 675–681.

Schwenke, D.C. *Lipoproteins, Oxidation and Atherogenesis.* Report of the Thirteenth Ross Conference on Medical Research.

USDA Nutrient Database. Accessed on line October 19, 1998.

www.diabetes.org., accessed October 19, 1998.

High Blood Pressure (Hypertension)

Brody, J. "A New Look at an Ancient Remedy: Celery." *New York Times,* June 9, 1992, page C-3.

http://nhlbi.nih.gov/nhlbi/nhlbi.htm, accessed June 16, 1998.

Morgan, B.L.G. *Nutrition Prescription.* New York: Crown Publishers, 1987.

Schardt, David. "Phytochemicals—Plants Against Cancer." *Nutrition Action Health Letter,* Center for Science in the Public Interest, Vol. 21. No. 3, April 1994.

www.amhrt.org, Heart & Stroke Guide, accessed June 16, 1998.

Human Papilloma Virus

Coll, D.A., et al. "Treatment of Recurrent Respiratory Papillomatosis with Indole-3-Carbinol." *American Journal of Otolaryngolgy* 18 (1997): 283–285.

Rosen, C.A., et al. "Preliminary Results of the Use of Indole-3 Carbinol for Recurrent Respiratory Papillomatosis." *Otolaryngology Head and Neck Surgery* 118(6) (June 1998): 10–15.

www.plannedparenthood.org, November 18, 1998.

Menopause

Clarke, R. "Estrogen, Phytoestrogens and Breast Cancer." AICR Annual Research Conference, August 31, 1995. Dietary Phytochemicals in Cancer Prevention and Treatment. Session III.

Dalais, F.S. "Soy and Menopause," *The Soy Connection,* Vol. 5, No. 4, Fall 1997.

Jacobs, D.R., et al. "Whole-Grain Intake May Reduce the Risk of Ischemic Heart Disease Death in Post Menopausal Women: The Iowa Women's Health Study." *American Journal of Clinical Nutrition* (1998): 48–57.

Jordan, C.V. "Designer Estrogens," *Scientific American* (October 1998): 60–67.

Knight, D.C., Eden, J.A. "A Review of the Clinical Effects of Phytoestrogens." *Obstetrics and Gynecology* 87(5) (May 1996).

Murkies, A.L., et al. "Dietary Flour Supplementation Decreases Post-Menopausal Hot Flushes: Effect of Soy and Wheat." *Maturitas* 21(3) (April 1995): 189–195.

Weed, S.S. *Menopausal Years, The Wise Woman Way.* Woodstock, New York: Ash Tree Publishing, 1992.

Wilcox, G., et al. "Oestrogenic Effects of Plant Foods in Postmenopausal Women." *British Medical Journal* 301 (Oct. 20, 1996).

Osteoporosis

"Avoiding the Fracture Zone." *Nutrition Action Health Letter* 25(3) (April 1998).

National Osteoporosis Foundation, *www.nof.org,* October 21, 1998.

Osteoporosis and Related Bone Disease, *http://www.osteo.org,* National Resource Center.

Proulx, W., Weaver, C.M. "Calcium Absorption from Plants." *The Soy Connection,* Vol. 2, No. 2.

Rose, D.P., Hatala, M.A. "Dietary Fatty Acids and Breast Cancer Invasion and Metastasis." *Nutrition and Cancer* 21(2) (1994): 103–111.

Wactawski-Wende, Jeanne. University of Buffalo, Presentation at the American Association for the Advancement of Science.

Wilcox, G., et al. "Oestrogenic Effects of Plant Foods in Postmenopausal Women." *British Medical Journal* 301 (Oct. 20, 1996).

www.nap.edu/books/0309063507/html/index.html.

Premenstrual Syndrome

"Human Disease and Disorders." In *Mayo Clinic Family Health Book,* William Morrow and Co. Inc., 1990, p. 1062.

Jacobs, S.T., et al. "Calcium Carbonate and the premenstrual syndrome: Effects on Premenstrual and Menstrual Symptoms." *American Journal of Obstetrics and Gynecology* 179 (1998): 444–452.

Jordan, C.V. "Designer Estrogens." *Scientific American* (October 1998): 60–67.

Kaufman, P.B., et al. "A Comparative Survey of Leguminous Plants as Sources of the Isoflavones, Genistein and Daidzein: Implications for Human Nutrition and Health." *The Journal of Alternative and Complementary Medicine* 3(1) (1997): 7–12.

Messina, M., Barnes, S. "The Role of Soy Products in Reducing Risk of Cancer." *Journal of the National Cancer Institute* 83(8) (1991): 541–545.

Northrup, C. *Women's Bodies, Women's Wisdom.* Bantam Books, 1994.

Wahlqvist, M.L., Dalais. "Phytoestrogens: Emerging Multifaceted Plant Compounds." *Medical Journal of Australia* 167 (Aug. 4, 1997): 119–120.

Additional References

Adler, A.J., and Holub, B.J. "Effect of Garlic and Fish-oil Supplementation on Serum Lipid and Lipoprotein Concentrations in Hypercholesterolemic Men." *American Journal of Clinical Nutrition* 65 (1997): 445–450.

Agarwal, R., et al. "Inhibitory Effect of Silymarin, an Anti-hepatoxic Flavonoid, on 12-o-Tetradecanoylphorbol-13-acetate Induced Epidermal Ornitine Carboxylase Activity and Mrna in Sencar Mice." *Carcinogenesis* 15(6) (1994): 1099–1103.

American Heart Association website: http// www.amhrt.org. Heart and stroke guide, accessed June 16, 1998.

The American Macular Degeneration Foundation: www.macular.org, accessed November 18, 1998.

Ames, Bruce N. "Dietary Carcinogens and Anticarcinogens." *Science,* 1983.

Anderson, J.W., B.M. Johnstone, and M.E. Cook-Newell. "Meta-Analysis of the Effects of Soy Protein Intake on Serum Lipids." *New England Journal of Medicine* 333 (1995): 276–282.

Aoki, T., et al. "Staphage Lysate and Lentinan as Immunoodulators and/or Immunopotentiators in Clinic and Experimental Systems." In *Augmenting Agents in Cancer Therapy,* ed. E.M. Hersh, et.al., pp. 101–112. New York: Raven Press, 1981.

Avila, M.A., et al. "Quercetin Mediates the Down-Regulation of Mutant p53 in the Human Breast Cancer Cell Line MDA-MB468." *Cancer Research* 54 (1994): 2424–2458.

Axelson, M., et al. "Origin of Lignans in Mammals and Identification of a Precursor from Plants." *Nature* 298(12) (1982): 659–660.

Ballister, B. *Fruit and Vegetable Stand.* Woodstock, NY: Overlook Press, 1985.

Barnes, S., and H. Kim. "Soy Isoflavones, Estrogens and Growth Factor Signaling." *The Soy Connection* 6(2) (1998).

Beardsley, Tim. "A War Not Won." *Scientific America* (January 1994): 130–138.

Berges, R.R., et al. "The B-Sitosterol Study Group Randomised, Placebo-Controlled, Double-Blind Clinical Trial of B-Sitosterol in Patients with Benign Prostatic Hyperplasia." *Lancet* 345 (1995): 1529–1532.

Block, E. "The Chemistry of Garlic and Onions." *Scientific American* 252 (1985): 114–119.

Bradlow, H. Leon. Personal communication, April 22, 1998, Strang Cornell Research Center for Breast Cancer Research.

———. Strang Cornell Research Labs, N.Y. Personal communication, July 21, 1995.

Brody, Jane. "Personal Health." *New York Times* (August 27, 1997).

———. "A New Look at an Ancient Remedy: Celery." *New York Times* (June 9, 1992), p. C3.

Calbom, Cherie, and Maureen Keane. *Juicing for Life*. Garden City Park, NY: Avery Publishing Group, 1992.

Caragay, A.B. "Cancer-Preventive Foods and Ingredients." *Food Technology* (4) (1992): 65–68.

Carter, J.P., et al. "Hypothesis: Dietary Management May Improve Survival from Nutritionally Linked Cancers Based on Analysis of Representative Cases." *Journal of the American College of Nutrition* 12(3) (1993): 209–226.

Chihara, G., et al. "Anti-tumor and Metastasis-inhibitory Activities of Lentinan as an Immunomodulator." *Cancer Detection and Prevention,* Supplement 1 (1987): 423–475.

Colbin, Annemarie. *Food and Healing*. New York: Ballantine Books, 1986.

Coll, D.A., et al. "Treatment of Recurrent Respiratory Papillomatosis with Indole-3-Carbinol." *American Journal of Otolaryngology* 18(4) (1997): 283–285.

Craig, W.J. "Phytochemicals: Guardians of Our Health." *Journal of the American Dietetic Association* (Supplement 2) (1997): S199–S204.

Crowell, Dr. Pamela, Professor of Biology at Purdue University at Indianapolis. Personal communication, November 6, 1997.

Crowell, P.L., S.A. Ayoubi, and Y.D. Burke. "Antitumorgenic Effects of Limonene and Perillyl Alcohol Against Pancreatic and Breast Cancer." *Dietary Phytochemicals in Cancer Prevention and Treatment*. New York: Pleneum Press, 1996.

Crowell, P.L., and M.N. Gould. "Chemoprevention and Therapy of Cancer by d-Limonene." *Critical Reviews in Oncogenesis* 5(1) (1994): 1–22.

Cunnane, S.C., et al. "High Alpha Linolenic Acid Flaxseed: Some Nutritional Properties in Humans." *British Journal of Nutrition* 69 (1993): 443–453.

Dalais, F.S. "Soy and Menopause." *The Soy Connection* 5(4) (1997).

Davidson, M.H., et al. "Long Term Effects of Consuming Foods Containing Psyllium Seed Husk on Serum Lipids in Subjects with Hypercholesterolemia." *American Journal of Clinical Nutrition* 67 (1998): 367–376.

Davis, D.L., et al. "Medical Hypothesis: Xenoestrogens as Preventable Causes of Breast Cancer." *Environmental Health Perspectives* 101 (1993): 372–377.

Deboles Company. Personal communication, November 16, 1998.

DiMasco-Murphy, M.E., and H. Sies. "Antioxidant Defense Systems: The Role of Carotenoids, Tocopherols and Thiols." *American Journal of Clinical Nutrition* 53 (1991): 194S–200S.

Djuric, Z., et al. "Oxidative DNA Damage Levels in Blood from Women at High Risk for Breast Cancer Are Associated with Dietary Intakes of Meats, Vegetables, and Fruits." *Journal of the American Dietetic Association* 98 (1998): 524–528.

Duke, Dr. James. Personal communication, January 30, 1998.

Elmer, G.W., C.M. Surawicz, and L.V. McFarland. "Biotherapeutic Agents." *Journal of the American Medical Association* 275 (11) (1996): 870–876.

Elson, C.E., and S.G. Yu. "The Chemoprevention of Cancer by Mevalonate-Derived Constituents of Fruits and Vegetables." *Journal of Nutrition* 124 (1994): 607–614.

Elson, Charles, University of Wisconsin at Madison. Personal communication, April 22, 1998.

Erdman, J.W., T.L. Bierer, and E.T. Gugger. "Absorption and Transport of Carotenoids: Carotenoids in Human Health." *Annals of the New York Academy of Sciences* 691 (1993): 76–85.

Erdman, J.W., and S.M. Potter. "Soy and Bone Health." *The Soy Connection* 5(2) (1997).

Fahey, J.W., et al. "Broccoli Sprouts: An Exceptionally Rich Source of Inducers of Enzymes That Protect Against Chemical Carcinogen." *Proceedings of the National Academy of Science* 94(9) (1997): 10367–10372.

Fiala, E.S., B.S. Reddy, and J.H. Weisburger. "Naturally Occurring Anticarcinogenic Substances in Foodstuffs." *Annual Reviews in Nutrition* 5 (1985): 295–321.

Folts, Dr. John D., University of Wisconsin Medical School. Presentation at the Conference of the American College of Cardiology, 1997.

"Food for Thought II," Report of Diet, Nutrition and Food Safety. International Food Information Council, February 1998.

Fotsis, T., et al. "Genistein, a Dietary Derived Inhibitor of In Vitro Angiogenesis." *Proceedings of the National Academy of Science* 90 (1993): 2690–2694.

Garg, Abhimanyu. "High Monounsaturated-fat Diets for Patients with Diabetes Mellitus: A Meta-analysis." *American Journal of Clinical Nutrition* 67 (supplement) (1998): 577S–582S.

Giovannucci, A.A., et al. "Intake of Carotenoids and Retinol in Relation to Risk of Prostate Cancer." *Journal of the National Cancer Institute* 87 (23) (1995): 1767–1776.

Glore, S.R., et al. "Soluble Fiber and Serum Lipids: A Literature Review." *Journal of the American Dietetics Association* 94 (1994): 425–436.

Goldbeck, David, and Nikki Goldbeck. *Nikki and David Goldbeck's American Wholefoods Cuisine*. New American Library, 1983.

Grabhorn, R. *Commonplace Book of Cookery*. San Francisco: North Point Press, 1985.

Greenwald, P. "Chemoprevention of Cancer." *Scientific American* (September 1996): 96.

Hecht, S.S., et al. "Effects of Watercress Consumption on Metabolism of a Tobacco-Specific Lung Carcinogen in Smokers," *Cancer Epidemiology, Biomarkers and Prevention* 4 (1995): 877–884.

Hecht, Steven S. American Health Foundation, Valhalla, N.Y. Personal communication, January 2, 1996.

Hohl, Raymond J. "Monoterpenes as Regulators of Malignant Cell Proliferation." *Dietary Phytochemicals in Cancer Prevention and Treatment* (1996): 137–149.

Hunt, S.M., and J.L. Groff. *Advanced Nutrition and Human Metabolism.* Boston: Thomson Learning, 1995.

Hunter, J. "Stalking Greens, Potherbs and Shoots." *Countryside and Small Stock Journal* 82(3) (1998): 59.

Hylton, William, ed. *The Rodale Herb Book.* Emmaus, PA: Rodale Press, 1976.

Imai, K., and K. Nakachi. " Cross Sectional Study of Effects of Drinking Green Tea on Cardiovascular and Liver Disease." *British Medical Journal* 310 (1995): 693–696.

Ip, C., and D.J. Lisk. "Enrichment of Selenium of Allium Vegetables for Cancer Prevention." *Carcinogenesis* 15(9) (1994): 1881–1885.

Jang, M., et al. "Antioxidant Defense Systems: The Role of Carotenoids, Tocopherols and Thiols." *American Journal of Clinical Nutrition* 53 (1991): 194S–200S.

———. "Cancer Chemopreventive Activity of Resveratrol, a Natural Product Derived from Grapes." *Science* (1997): 275.

Jankun, J., et al. "Why Drinking Green Tea Could Prevent Cancer." *Nature* 387 (1997): 561.

Jordan, C.V. "Designer Estrogens." *Scientific American* (October 1998): 60–67.

Kaufman, P.B., et al. "A Comparative Survey of Leguminous Plants as Sources of the Isoflavones, Genistein and Daidzein: Implications for Human Nutrition and Health." *Journal of Alternative and Complementary Medicine* 3(1) (1997): 7–12.

Kelly, G.S. "Bromelain: A Literature Review and Discussion of Its Therapeutic Applications." *Alternative Medicine Reviews* 1(4) (1996): 243–257.

Kennedy, A.R., et al. "Suppression of Carcinogenesis in the Intestines of Min Mice in the Soybean Derived Bowman-Birk Inhibitor." *Cancer Research* 56 (1996): 679.

Kensler, T.W., et al. "Mechanism of Protection Against Afltoxin Tumorgenicity in Rats Fed 5-(2-Pyranzinyl)-4-methyl-1,2-dithiol-3-thione (Oltipraz) and Related 1,2Dithiol-3-thiones and 1,2-Dithiolethiones." *Cancer Research* 4 (1987): 4271–4277.

Khechai, F., et al. "Effect of Advanced Glycation End Product-Modified Albumin on Tissue Factor Expression by Monocytes; Role of Oxidant Stress and Protein Tyrosine Kinase Activation." *Arteriosclerosis, Thrombosis, and Vascular Biology* 17 (11) (1997): 2885–2890.

Knight, D.C., and J.A. Eden. "A Review of the Clinical Effects of Phytoestrogens." *Obstetrics and Gynecology* 87(5) Part 2 (1996): 897–904.

Kurowska, E.M. "Soy and Reduced Risk of Cardiovascular Disease." *The Soy Connection* 59(3) (1997).

Kushi, A. *Complete Guide to Macrobiotic Cooking.* New York: Warner Books, 1985.

The Kushi Institute website: *http://www.macrobiotics.org,* accessed October 21, 1997.

Leaf, A., and P.C. Weber. "Cardiovascular Effects of n-3 Fatty Acids." *New England Journal of Medicine* 318(9) (1988): 549–556.

Leiberman, Shari. *The Real Vitamin and Mineral Book.* Garden City Park, N.Y: Avery Publishing Group, Inc., 1997.

Leibman, B. "The Whole Grain Guide." *Nutrition Action Health Letter* 24 (2) (1997).

Leibman, Bonnie. "Beyond Beta-Carotene." *Nutrition Action Health Letter* 22 (1) (1995).

Mandell, G.L., J.E. Bennet, and R. Dolin. *Mandell, Douglas, and Bennett's Principles and Practice of Infectious Diseases.* Philadelphia: Churchill Livingstone, 1995.

Mangels, A.R., et al. "Carotenoid Content of Fruits and Vegetables: An Evaluation of Analytic Data." *Journal of the American Dietetic Association* 93 (1993): 284–296.

Mares-Perlman, J.A., et al. "Serum Anti-Oxidants and Age-Related Macular Degeneration in a Population-Based Case Control Study." *Archives of Ophthalmology* (1995): 113.

Messina, M. "Soy Shows Promise in Slowing Prostate Cancer Rate of Growth." *The Soy Connection* 6(4) (1998).

Messina, M., and S. Barnes. "The Role of Soy Products in Reducing Cancer." *Cancer Prevention and Control* 83(8) (1991).

Michnovicz, J.J., and H.L. Bradlow. "Altered Estrogen Metabolism and Excretion in Humans Following Consumption of Indole-3-Carbinol." *Nutrition and Cancer* 16 (1991): 59–66.

Mindell, E. *Earl Mindell's Soy Miracle.* Fireside Books, 1995.

Mooradian, A.S., et al. "Selected Vitamins and Minerals in Diabetes." *Diabetes Care* 17 (5) (1994).

Morgan, Brian L.G. *Nutrition Prescription.* New York: Crown Publishing, 1987.

Morse, M.A., et al. "Inhibition of 4(methylnitrosamino)-1-3pyridyl)-1 Butanone Induced DNA Adduct Formation and Tumorgenicity in the Lung of F344 Rats by Dietary Phenethyl Isothiocynate." *Cancer Research* 49 (1989): 549–553.

Muktar, H., S.K. Katiyar, and R. Agarwal. "Cancer Chemoprevention by Green Tea Components." In *Diet and Cancer: Markers, Prevention, and Treatment,* 1992 Conference on Diet and Cancer. New York: Plenum Press, 1994.

Muktar, Hasan. "Polyphenol Phytochemical Content of Green Tea and Artichokes." Address at the Conference on Dietary Phytochemicals in Cancer Prevention and Treatment, August 31 and September 1, 1995.

Murkies, A.L., et al. "Dietary Flour Supplementation Decreases Post-Menopausal Hot Flushes: Effect of Soy and Wheat." *Maturitas* 21(3) (1995): 189–195.

Nash, M. "Stopping a Killer in Its Track." *Time Magazine,* April 25, 1994.

National Heart, Lung and Blood Institute: *http://nhlbi.nih.gov/nhlbi/nhlbi.html.*

National Osteoporosis Foundation: *http:// www.nof.org.*

Newmark, H.L. "Plant Phenolics as Potential Cancer Prevention Agents." Dietary Phytochemicals in Cancer Prevention and Treatment. AICR, Plenum Press: N.Y., 1996.

Newmark, Harold. Speaker at Conference August 31, and September 1, 1995. "Dietary Phytochemicals in Cancer Prevention and Treatment."

Noble, H.B. "A Handful of Nuts and a Healthier Heart." *New York Times.* November 17, 1998.

Northrup, Christiane, M.D. *Women's Bodies, Women's Wisdom.* New York: Bantam Books, 1994.

Oesterling, J.E. "Benign Prostatic Hyperplasia Medical and Minimally Invasive Treatment." *New England Journal of Medicine* 332(2) (1995).

Osteoporosis and Related Bone Disease-National Resource Center: *http://www.osteo.org*.

Pawlak, Laura. *A Perfect Ten: Phyto "New-Trients" Against Cancers*. Emeryville, Calif.: Biomed General Corp., 1998

Peterson, J., and Dwyer, J. "Taxonomic Classification Helps Identify Flavonoid Containing Foods on a Semiquantitative Food Frequency Questionnaire." *Journal of the American Dietetic Association* 98 (1998): 677–682, 685.

Pinto, John. "Phytochemicals and Cancer." Presentation to the Mid Hudson Dietetics Association, April 8, 1998.

Planned Parenthood website: *www.plannedparenthood.org*, accessed November 18, 1998.

"The Position Paper of the American Dietetic Association: Phytochemicals and Functional Foods." *Journal of the American Dietetic Association* 95 (4) (1995): 493–496.

Potter, John, Dr. Personal communication, May 8, 1996.

Potter, S.M. "Overview of Proposed Mechanisms for the Hypocholesterolemic Effect of Soy." *Journal of Nutrition* 125 (1995): 606S–611S.

Pronsky, Z.M. *Powers and Moore's Food Medications Interactions,* 9th ed. Pottstown, PA: Food Medications Interactions, 1995.

Proulx W., and C.M. Weaver. "Calcium Absorption from Plants." *The Soy Connection* 2 (2).

Reaven, P. "Dietary and Pharmacologic Regimens to Reduce Lipid Oxidation in Non-Insulin Dependent Diabetes Mellitus." *American Journal of Clinical Nutrition* 62 (1995): 1483S–1489S.

Rimm, E.B., et al. "Folate and Vitamin B_6 Status from Diet and Supplements in Relation of Risk in Coronary Heart Disease Among Women." *Journal of the American Medical Association* 279(5) 1998: 359–364.

Rose, D.P., and M.A. Hatala. "Dietary Fatty Acids and Breast Cancer Invasion and Metastasis." *Nutrition and Cancer* 21(2) (1994): 103–111.

Rose, D.R. "Dietary Fatty Acids and Cancer." *American Journal of Clinical Nutrition* 66 (supplement) (1997): 998S–1003S.

Rose, J. *Herbs and Things*. New York: Perigee Books, 1983.

Rosen, C.A., et al. "Preliminary Results of the Use of Indole-3 Carbinol for Recurrent Respiratory Papillomatosis." *Otolaryngology Head and Neck Surgery* 118(6) (1998): 810–815.

Rumessen, J., et al. "Fructans of Jerusalem Artichokes: Intestinal Transport, Absorption, Fermentation and Influence on Blood Glucose, Insulin and C-peptide Responses in Healthy Subjects." *American Journal of Clinical Nutrition* 52 (1990): 675–681.

Salmi, H.A., and S. Sarna. "Effect of Silymarin on Chemical, Functional and Morphological Alterations of the Liver." *Scandinavian Journal of Gastroenterology* 17 (1982): 517–521.

Schardt, D. "Phytochemicals—Plants Against Cancer." *Nutrition Action Health Letter* 21(3) (1994).

Schardt, D., and B. Leibman. "Garlic vs. Garlic." *Nutrition Action Health Letter* 22(6) (1995).

Schardt, D., and Schmidt. "Garlic: Clove at First Sight?" *Nutrition Action Health Letter* 22(6) (1995).

Schelp, F.P., and P. Pongpaew. "Protection Against Cancer Through Nutritionally Induced Increase of Endogenous Proteinase Inhibitors—A Hypothesis." *International Journal of Epidemiology* 17(2) (1988).

Schulze, J., A. Malone, and E. Richter. "Intestional Metabolism of 4-(methylnitrosamino-1-(3-pyridyl)1-butanone in Rats: Sex-Difference, Inductibility and Inhibition by Phenethylisothiocyanate." *Carcinogenesis* 16 (1995): 1733–1740.

Schwenke, D.C. "Lipoproteins, Oxidation and Atherogenesis." Report of the Thirteenth Ross Conference on Medical Research.

Seddon, J.M., et al. "Dietary Carotenoids, Vitamin A, C, and E and Advanced Age-Related Macular Degeneration." *Journal of the American Medical Association* 2723(18) (1994): 1413–1420.

Simopoulos, A.P., et al. "Common Purslane: A Source of Omega-3 Fatty Acids and Antioxidants." *Journal of the American College of Nutrition* (H51) 11(4) (August 1992): 374–382.

Spiegel, J.E., et al. "Safety and Benefits of Fructooligosaccharides as Food Ingredients." *Food Technology* (January 1994).

Spiller, G. Presentation at the American Heart Association's 36th Annual Conference on Cardiovascular Disease Epidemiology and Prevention. March 15, 1997.

Stacey, M. "The Rise and Fall of Kilmer McCully." *The New York Times Magazine* (August 10, 1997): 25.

Stein, Jess, ed. *The Random House Dictionary of the English Language*. New York: Random House, 1968.

Steinmetz, K.A., and J.D. Potter. "Vegetables, Fruit, and Cancer: II Mechanisms." *Cancer, Causes and Control* 2 (1991): 427–442.

Steinmetz, K.A., et al. "Vegetables, Fruit and Colon Cancer in the Iowa's Women's Health Study." *The American Journal of Epidemiology* 139(1) (1994).

Sugiyama, K. "Dietary Eritadenine Modifies Plasma Phosphatidylcholine Molecular Species Profile in Rats Fed Different Types of Fat." *Journal of Nutrition* 127 (1997): 593–599.

Thoreau, Henry David. *Walden or Life in the Woods*. Mount Vernon, NY: Peter Pauper Press.

Thys-Jacobs, S., et al. "Calcium Carbonate and the Premenstrual Syndrome: Effects on Premenstrual Symptoms." *American Journal of Obstetrics and Gynecology* 179(2) (1998): 444–452.

Tiwari, R.K., et al. "Selective Responsiveness of Human Breast Cancer Cells to Indole-3-Carbinol, a Chemopreventive Agent." *Journal of the National Cancer Institute* 86(2) (1994): 126–131.

The Tomato Research Council. Notes from International Symposium on the Role of Lycopene and Tomato Products in Disease Prevention Given. March 3, 1997.

Uckun, F.M., et al. "Biotherapy of B-Cell Precursor Leukemia by Targeting Genistein to CD-19 Associated Tyrosine Kinases." *Science* 267 (1995).

USDA Nutrient Database for Standard Reference: *http://www.nal.usda.gov.*

"Veggies in a Pill." *Women's Health Advocate Newsletter* 5(4) (1998): 1–2, 8.

"Vitamins and Minerals, What to Take." *Nutrition Action Health Letter* (May 1998).

Wactawski-Wende, Jeanne, Ph.D., University of Buffalo. Presentation at the American Association for the Advancement of Science.

Wallis, C. "Curing Cancer—The Hype and the Hope." *Time Magazine* (May 18, 1998): 38–50.

Wang, H., and P. Murphy. "Isoflavone Content in Commercial Soybean Foods." *Journal of Agricultural and Food Chemistry* 42(8) (1994): 1666–1673.

Wattenberg, L.W. "Inhibition of Carcinogenesis by Minor Dietary Constituents." *Cancer Research* 52 (supplement) (1992): 2085S–2091S.

Weed, S.S. *Menopausal Years, The Wise Woman Way.* Woodstock, NY: Ash Tree Publishing, 1992.

Weil, Dr. Andrew. "Botanical Medicine in Modern Clinical Practice." Minutes of a meeting held at Columbia University College of Physicians and Surgeons, May 13–17, 1996.

Whitney, E.N., and E.M.N. Hamilton. *Understanding Nutrition.* Pymble, NSW, Australia: West Publishing Company, 1987.

Wilcox, G., et al. "Oestrogenic Effects of Plant Foods in Postmenopausal Women." *British Medical Journal* 301 (1996): 905.

Yu, Sha, et. al. "Anti-Tumor Activity of the Crude Saponins Obtained from Asparagus." *Cancer Letters* 104 (1996): 31–36.

Zheng, G., et al. "Chemoprevention of Benzo(a)pyrene-Induced Forestomach Cancer in Mice by Natural Phthalides from Celery Seed Oil." *Nutrition and Cancer* 19 (1993): 77–86.

Zheng, G.Q., P.M. Kenney, and L.K.T. Lam. "Anethofuran, Carvone and Limonene: Potential Cancer Chemopreventive Agents from Dill Weed Oil and Caraway Oil." *Planta Medica* 58 (1992): 338–341.

Index

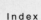